Who Cares

a memoir about caregiving and
coping with dementia

Anna Strosser

WHO CARES

a memoir about caregiving and coping with dementia

Copyright @2018 by Anna Strosser

ISBN: 978-1-54394-521-8 eBook: 978-1-54394-522-5
Editor: Margie Strosser

Cover Photo: Margie Strosser
Chair Drawing: Anna Strosser

mcdonoughpress.com
McDonough Press
P.O. Box 54402
Philadelphia, PA 19148

ACKNOWLEDGEMENTS

I want to thank my daughter Margie Strosser for her invaluable help and support in the writing and editing of this book. She also took the photographs of our later life. I could not have written the book without the encouragement of our Blue Eyed Irish American Writers Group (BEIAWG), consisting of Margie, my son Ed Strosser, our friend Jack Higgins, and occasionally Jack Strosser, my grandson. We have been meeting almost monthly for four years. Together we span four generations and 72 years in age. Even when it was hard for me to believe that I would actually be able to finish this book, they encouraged me to not give up.

I also owe a debt of gratitude to Jax Lowell for carefully reading an earlier draft, and sharing many insightful notes.

Most of all I want to thank my husband Ken, who has kept me engaged throughout our lives together, as we sifted through the mystery of his identity.

PREFACE

This book began as a story about my husband Ken, who is ninety-one years old and suffers from Vascular Dementia. As the book evolved it has become more about me, about living my life and making hard decisions. I have used my knowledge as a mother, a psychiatric nurse, an art therapist as well as a loving wife to provide meaning and satisfaction in a life diminished by confusion and memory loss. Most of all, my story is about a way to care for our loved ones within the extended family structure; a choice that benefits all concerned in ways that I could not have imagined when Ken and I set out on our journey.

Ken and I now live with our daughter Margie and son-in-law Edwin in a large row house in close-knit South Philadelphia, a long established ethnic neighborhood. Ken has a good pension and we both have Social Security so we are able to contribute to the house expenses. I am eighty-eight, have arthritis and a heart condition, which are manageable. I do some of the cooking and most of the laundry for the family. I manage steps well and take the subway to play bridge and go to art classes at least twice a week.

I am writing from the perspective of how Ken is functioning now in October 2014. He was not expected to live after a massive heart attack that he suffered about thirteen years ago in late 2001.

In this book I draw upon a chaotic childhood environment. I also needed to look at how my life as a psychiatric nurse helped me cope with Dementia. For years I kept notes and wrote in my journal. With the help of the writing group that Margie, our daughter, initiated I have been able to see some patterns and some of the emotional roadblocks I encountered along the way. I have tried to describe the changes I have gone through in the challenge of being an older caregiver, while taking care of myself as well.

Ken is a person who did not like arguments, kept his temper under control and rarely made demands of others, including our children and me. I always had plans, but was usually in the dark about what Ken thought of them. Although he seldom disagreed with me, I often felt guilty because I made the decisions. I was never sure if he was afraid of making the decisions or feared the consequences if he was wrong. Sometimes he would resolve problems by distancing himself from them. When it involved the children I didn't disagree with him. He always helped to resolve things.

There is a great deal of confusion about the differences between the various forms of deterioration of cognitive ability in older people amongst both the medical profession and families with members who are affected. Dementias are often thought of in the popular culture as 'senility' or 'senile dementia' which reflects the false belief that serious mental decline is part and parcel with natural aging, which is not necessarily true. The terms Dementia, Alzheimer's, Vascular Dementia, and Mild Cognitive Impairment (MCI) are often used interchangeably but are in fact have very different causes, conditions, and the course they take as the disease progresses.

Dementia is a general term for the decline in mental ability severe enough to interfere with daily life.

Alzheimer's Disease is the most common type of Dementia and accounts for 69-80% of cases of Dementia in the United States, according to the Alzheimer's Association. In Alzheimer's Disease cognition declines as the effected brain cells gradually die. Memory loss gradually worsens and other symptoms may emerge, such as language difficulty, impairment of judgment and mood changes.

Vascular Dementia is a form of Dementia that is characterized by memory loss and impaired judgment, language and social behavior. Vascular Dementia can occur quite suddenly or progress slowly over time, and is directly correlated with blood pressure, age, and cardiovascular complications. It describes a group of symptoms severely affecting intellectual and social abilities which interfere with daily functioning, difficulty carrying out complex tasks and mood or personality changes.

The most common form of Vascular Dementia is characterized by short- term memory impairment, a symptom from which Ken continues to suffer. Other cognitive areas such as language use and processing speed may be only slightly and unnoticeably affected.

The most prominent changes are seen in executive functioning and include problems with thinking, walking and performing everyday activities. Many people with Vascular Dementia suffer from depression, which can result in less motivation to continue their usual activities, or lack of interest in the world around them.

The lack of memory for events and people can make the individual extremely anxious about daily life. Tasks that used to be routine, can now seem overwhelming due to apathy or lack of initiation.

Recent research assumes that a full two-thirds of Dementia sufferers are taken care of in their own home or in the homes of their families. No matter the cause, Dementia be quite challenging for a caregiver.

In 2014, I received the following letter from Alice, a long-time friend. I believe Alice poignantly speaks for many of the individuals and families who are struggling to under-stand and find ways to deal effectively with Dementia.

> *Dear Anna,*
>
> *I had a very hard time while my husband suffered with Dementia. I hope you don't have what I had. He could never be left alone; he would fall, get out of the house and then fall. He broke his arm on one of these outings and never could use it again it was so badly crushed. Then he could not bathe himself, shower himself or comb his hair. I had to cut up his food and then he was taught to eat left-handed.*

I washed every night, as he could not always make it to the bathroom. He didn't recognize our children or grandkids, so we made a book with their pictures in it and their names and we would show it to him to try to refresh his memory. That never worked either. Going to a support group helped me some but I never had outside help. I was the sole care-giver. It was a hard time for me for seven long years. He didn't want anyone else to stay with him if I went out. He gave them a hard time. Even though he didn't know who I was, he still wanted me there. He wasn't good with my three children either.

It is a very debilitating disease and the entire family is affected. we never know what he might say. Most of our friends stopped coming around. That was hard and embarrassing for me.

I will write again,
Love, Alice

This book is my way of reaching out to those caregivers, like my friend Alice and myself, who need to hear stories that help them learn to cope and find common-sense ways of managing that are successful and rewarding to everyone involved.

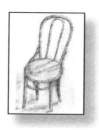

CHAPTER ONE...1

CHAPTER TWO 11

CHAPTER THREE 25

CHAPTER FOUR 39

CHAPTER FIVE 49

CHAPTER SIX 57

CHAPTER SEVEN...65

CHAPTER EIGHT 75

CHAPTER NINE 87

CHAPTER TEN 103

COPING: A QUICK LIST 115

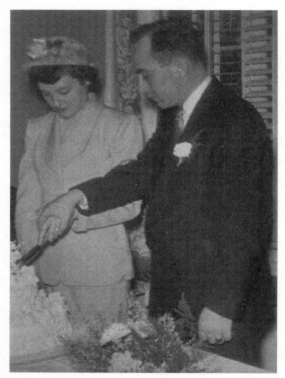

Anna and Ken on their wedding day
Pittsburgh January, 1951

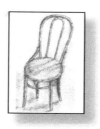

CHAPTER ONE

I knew that I had looked attractive the evening I first saw Ken in 1950. I'd worn the navy blue suit that I'd just finished paying for and a light blue blouse with a ruffled collar that framed my face. In the hope of meeting somebody exciting, I was not wearing my glasses. This was the era of Dorothy Parker's famous decree, "Men seldom make passes at girls who wear glasses." And I believed it meant never; not seldom.

So when the phone call came the next day I was ecstatic.

"I saw you across the room at the Catholic Club meeting last night," the voice said. "I'm Ken Strosser and my brother Larry knows your sister and gave me your telephone number." He asked me if I would go out with him and I agreed with only a little apprehension. After all, it was the Catholic Club and his brother knew Mary. What could be more appropriate?

Our first date was almost the last one. He agreed to meet me at a place that we both knew, Schenley Park, in Pittsburgh. I was wearing navy blue again, a dress with a full skirt and an attached red and white striped petticoat which flashed in and out when I moved, red shoes with a strap across the instep and a red jacket.

I waited patiently for about half an hour and had decided to get on the next bus and go home when he showed up, out of breath and apologizing for being late. I just looked at him and moved toward the arriving bus.

"Please stay," he said. But those tempting blue eyes, the black hair in the short, military haircut, his sad look as he apologized profusely, won me over. I didn't even see the bus pass by.

It was a lovely spring day; the leaves still had that fresh, light green look of spring. We strolled past the stage where summer concerts would be held in another month. I didn't mind that Ken was quiet. But I was still a little annoyed with his late arrival and didn't want to admit it.

"Oh look," I finally said, "there's a playground." I ran toward it, swishing my skirt as I ran. After years of wartime drab dresses and re-soled shoes, the New Look – full skirts and petticoats – were in style, and I was too. Ken caught up with me and we sat on the swings and talked about ourselves.

I had finished nurses' training three years earlier and was working at St. Margaret's Hospital in Pittsburgh. Ken had graduated from college at the same time with a degree in Metallurgy and was working for Wood Works, a research office for the United States Steel Corporation nearby in McKeesport, Pennsylvania. I worked the evening shift, 3pm to 11pm, and lots of ti.mes Ken would pick me up and drive me home.

The first weekend that I was free from work at St. Margaret's, just three weeks after we met, we drove to Mercer, a small farm town in Western Pennsylvania, to meet his family. His parents Walter and Lucille, three of his four brothers and his sister were there. All I remember about that visit was that I felt good in the black skirt and white pique blouse that I was wearing, and the fact that his mother filled the dinner plates and passed them around as if we were in a restaurant.

That summer was a kaleidoscope of sun and sand, music and laughter and colors and new places; just getting in a car was exciting after a lifetime of streetcars. Invariably Ken would say: "An ice cream shop coming up!" We stopped at ice cream stands in all of Western Pennsylvania, satisfying Ken's love for the confection. His love for me was becoming obvious too. Sometimes we went to the beach at Lake Erie and spent the day gorging on ice cream and hamburgers and lying on a blanket talking about what we liked about each other and exchanging sandy kisses. By the end of the summer, for the first time in my life, I was completely happy. I thought of nothing and nobody but Ken.

He surprised me one Saturday by taking me to a nightclub where Tony Bennett was starring. I was completely impressed, not just by his spending so much money, but because I could see how he loved the music. I never thought about music before except as a rhythm to dance to, but he gave his whole attention to it. We danced and argued with each other about the right way to turn in a polka, and about how wonderful Tony Bennett was while I thought about how wonderful Ken was. We first talked about marriage, but there was never any big declaration or question like "Will you marry me?" until that fall of 1950 when the rumor circulated among the St. Margaret's Hospital staff that any nurse in the Cadet Nurse Corp would be sent to Korea.

I was a Cadet Nurse. My Irish family was poor, and the opportunities for college scholarships were few. So when I graduated from high school in 1944 I joined the Cadet Nurse Corps Program. After America entered World War II, the demand for nurses increased dramatically. The United States Public Health Service established the Cadet Nurse Corps in response to the shortage. Nursing students like me were promised free training with pay, room and board, and uniforms. I began my training at St. Joseph's Hospital on the South Side of Pittsburgh in 1944, the third year of the war. Even though it was not, strictly speaking, a military program, Cadet Nurses were required to serve in government service for several years after the war was over.

Even though there was no confirmation of the rumor that Cadet Nurses would be shipped off to serve in Korea, Ken and I decided to get married the following January, just in case it was true. I would have been eager to have gone six months before, but going to Korea was not the excitement I wanted at that point in my life.

We went to a Catholic Club Thanksgiving dance and I think of that as our engagement party. During the last dance he whispered in my ear "How about a wedding in January?". I felt like shouting YES, but settled on a whispered "Oh yes".

We were too excited to pay attention to the weather forecast that night and walked out of the club into more than a foot of snow. We made it out of the parking lot in the car, and as long as the streets were level we made progress. But my family's house was on one of the steepest hills in a city full of steep hills, and at some point the car really got stuck and we had to walk the rest of the way. I was wearing sandals and by the time we got home, even though Ken tried to keep me warm by almost carrying me up the hill, I was shivering with the cold and my feet felt frozen.

It was the worst snowstorm in Pittsburgh for many years to come. The mayor asked for volunteers to help clear the streets and Ken spent the next two days shoveling snow. I spent them in bed with a cold.

We decided to get married on January 27, 1951, with a simple wedding – just our families and a few friends at our catholic church, The Annunciation, on the north side of Pittsburgh. I don't remember walking down the aisle. I'm sure my father was with me, and my mother prepared the wedding breakfast which we celebrated in our dining room at home. My mind was in a fog. It was so hard to believe that I was getting married that not much registered except what I wore: a brand new beige suit and a hat with a narrow brim covered with flowers. New clothes had become very important to me. I had worn hand-me-downs, or welfare clothes, or a catholic school uniform my whole life, and I think by this time I was starved for beautiful clothes.

Before the wedding, Ken surprised me by suggesting that instead of going on a honeymoon we use the money for a down payment on a house. I had never heard of anybody buying a house when they got married. I thought people lived in apartments and sometime along the way might be able to buy a house – if they ever had the money.

When I was growing up houses were a painful part of the conversation in our family. My mother had bought our house on Charles Street in the late 1920s with money she earned by keeping a rooming house. During the Great Depression in the 1930s, she lost it to the "damnbankers", and then had to pay rent for the house that we still lived in. Every time she went to the real estate office to pay the rent, we heard about "her" house. So to me, a house was something so valuable that it was hard to believe it would really happen. This is a fundamental belief that has informed my whole life. To me a house is safe harbor; a place where I can weather storms, where I can be myself. I am in some sense a 'homebody', and every house I have lived in has been a deep part of my identity.

Looking back, I think that buying a house reflected a yearning for security for Ken. He had what, in those days, was a secure lifetime job as a metallurgical engineer, and having a house was part of his plan. For me, the plan was marrying him; the future would take care of itself. I loved him and knew I could trust him. He had all the qualities that my father lacked. Ken was smart too, but he used his brain to accomplish things and he had a sense of humor. Also he was handsome and he loved me. Well, my father was handsome and loved me too, but he was an alcoholic and Ken didn't drink. Daddy had more of a sense of humor than my mother, but the whiskey kept it hidden most of the time.

We spent two days in Washington DC after the wedding, but our real honeymoon was in a small apartment near where Ken worked in McKeesport while we were looking for a house. I had always lived in Pittsburgh, but Ken was raised in a small country town. When we talked about where to look for a house,

I think it never occurred to him to buy in the city. I was still in a dream state, and happy to go wherever he wanted.

We bought a house in Monroeville, a scattered farming community which was destined to become one of the fastest growing suburbs of Pittsburgh. Western Pennsylvania is a beautiful area and on our first visit to see the almost-finished house it was nestled near an orchard, a magic vision of tree after tree filled with white peach blossoms. Ken slowed the car and we crept along for the length of a city block, both of us speechless.

The house was red brick, set back from the road and surrounded by tall cherry trees with dark trunks that whispered to each other even with very little wind. The sight of those lovely trees added to the dream that I felt I was living.

This was a new world; the war was over, the depression was over, people had jobs, were making money and the government was underwriting low interest rates for veterans. We did what a great many other veterans families were doing. We bought a house in one of the new suburbs, which became even more popular than the New Look.

The neighborhood rapidly filled with young married veterans and little children. The husbands all worked at some distance. These were the 1950s - light years from the consciousness-raising sixties - so the wives stayed home, gossiped about each other, played bridge, and led otherwise seemingly aimless lives. Many of them had worked in various jobs during the war but now that the men were back seemed to accept that their place was in the home being only the housewife.

I wasn't good at being aimless. I had been brought up to think gossip was abhorrent and I was not a very good bridge player. Also, many of the men apparently were in positions where they made more money than Ken did, so I assumed that their wives felt more comfortable than I did not working. So, after our first child Margie was about two years old I started to work in a doctor's office two evenings a week and sometimes on Saturday. I had developed a plan for my life. When I worked at the hospital I had seen so many old and bitter nurses that I vowed I would stay in nursing until it became hard to do the nursing work with compassion. I would work as a nurse until it became a routine, uninteresting job. I would develop my interest in painting and writing, further my education, and eventually find work more compatible with my interests and my need for independence.

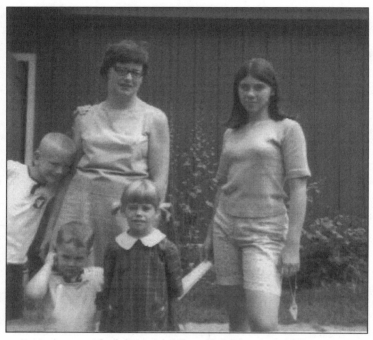

*Anna with (left to right) Jim, Ed, Terry, and Margie
Vandergrift August, 1966*

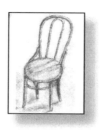

CHAPTER TWO

In the late 1950s or early 1960s the steel mills started slowing down. Countries that had been devastated during the war were building new, more efficient mills and selling steel at better prices. The metallurgy lab where Ken worked laid off workers, and Ken was transferred to the Cold Rolling Mill in the small town of Vandergrift, tucked into the Appalachian foothills, twenty five miles from the suburb where we were living.

Ken became a supervisor for production of carbon steel and worked shifts. He was more successful there than he had been at McKeesport, where his main job had been to write quality control reports. The men at the Vandergrift mill liked him and he worked well with them, and he stayed there for the next twenty-five years.

Ken was always a peaceful, non-confrontational person. He didn't like fighting or violence, he did not even go hunting when he was young even though everybody else did, including his father and brothers. In Ken's hometown, hunting was so much a way of life that students were even given official time off from school to go out into the woods and shoot. So, I think Ken's natural easy-going ways were not so easily accepted in a family of boys, nor in a man's world.

Being non-confrontational also meant that he invariably kept his temper in control and rarely made demands of me or others. The men in the mill liked him as a supervisor; he was cheerful, considerate and apparently consulted them about needed decisions. I found this out at parties which were held once a year for the employees. During the war he had been in the Navy, in charge of a Landing Craft Tank, an LCT, an amphibious assault ship for landing tanks on beachheads. As the ensign, Ken was in charge of actually constructing the ship from a 'kit' they were issued in San Francisco, and then slowly making their way across the Pacific in a flotilla that never saw combat and survived a typhoon. He told me once that he ran the ship the same way he did the mill floor, and it worked.

Ken never liked to talk about himself. When I tried to get him to do so, he politely refused. I never knew what he thought about most things, and he went along with most suggestions. So I was often unsure whether he liked an idea or not. But he was, and is, a truly loving husband. He was always there to hold me, to help me when I needed him. We had both knew loneliness and understood that about each other. Neither of us ever wanted to be lonely again, and I believe that is partly what has kept us together all of these years.

My parents were Irish immigrants. My father, John, was an alcoholic and was absent from home for long periods of time after I was about eight years old. My mother, Bridget, was a strict and devout Catholic. The only way my parents were able to express their feelings was by fighting, or leaving for long periods of time as my Dad did, "spending all our money on drink with those bums at the saloon", as my mother used to say. I was the third of six children, and we often related to each other in the same way as our parents did – fighting or running away. I always had a book nearby and could run to the attic and read. If it was summer, I sat in our vestibule. There was a large inner door with a glass panel inside two large wooden doors to the street. I would sit behind it, leave one of the wooden ones open for air and swat the flies while I read.

Both Ken and I came from large families. Ken's father was a World War I veteran and worked as a rural postman. His mother stayed home. Because Ken was considered smart he was sent to school early, when he was five years old. He studied hard, anxious about doing everything right, a trait which carried over into his adult life.

After spending time with his family, I realized that the ordinary communication among his siblings was telling jokes, sometimes inconsiderate of feelings, or talking about sports. Most of this was conducted by his four more vocal brothers. Larry, the oldest, seemed to be the leader. Ken was next to Larry in age and they were friends. None of them, it seemed, were comfortable expressing their emotions or feelings directly. And Ken was solidly part of his family in this regard.

Ken was very good with the children, paid attention to them. Margie was bright and cheerful, full of ideas and energy. Jim, our second child, had a lively personality too and was curious about everything he came in contact with, a lifetime characteristic. I found it hard being the ogre, which I often was. I felt like I had to control everything, so I never did figure out whether I seized control in our relationship, or if he simply allowed me to because I sounded so determined.

Ken could never tolerate unhappy children. If they cried he had to soothe them somehow; he would do anything to stop it, or get away from it. This became a problem as they grew older, especially with our youngest daughter, Terry, who was born in 1962. She was extremely hard to control, and screamed a lot when she was a baby.

Terry seemed to have something inside her mind that at times imprisoned her joyful spirit. As she got older, she tried hard to do what she had been told was the right way to act, but when she failed she became almost hysterical. Music was very soothing for her but she got furious if interrupted when she was listening to it. She seemed almost obsessively orderly; the food had to be precisely arranged on her plate, it was often cold before she could eat it. When she was very little she carried all of her toys around the house with her in a large box. When she was about ten or eleven she often slept on top of the bedcover for fear of disarranging it.

I knew that something was wrong and she and I needed help. When I consulted school psychologists I was told by them that I was a poor mother, and Terry merely needed more discipline. We had adopted her when she was two months old through

Catholic Charities, and they had no help to offer me. They had no health history for her, only that Terry had been left in a hospital nursery for two months after her birth. Catholic Charities had a strict confidentiality agreement with her birth mother, and refused to give us any more information. Unfortunately, I believed them.

Now when I look back on that time, I grieve that I did not know how to get more legal help to extract the information about Terry's family that we needed so badly. I felt that there was no one to share my worries about my daughter; I became frustrated about my inability to get the help I knew she needed. Terry was eventually diagnosed as being hyperactive, which wasn't much help because nobody, including principals, teachers, doctors and psychologists, seemed to know what to do about it. Terry's demands were great, and Ken would often give in to her because her behavior was so disturbing and upsetting to him.

The amount of time spent on our daughter Terry's needs had its effect on the whole family. Our other children – Margie, Jim, and our youngest son Ed - resented it but they seemed to be able to function fairly well in spite of it. I could usually control her behavior in some ways at home by keeping her close to me and sometimes holding her for hours. But once she got away from me she took off like an exploded missile. For a short time Ritalin seemed to help but the doctors were so uncertain about its long-term effects at the time that the pediatrician refused to order subscriptions for it after about a year. We were lucky to have a kindergarten teacher who was older, calm and able to handle her much as I did.

When Terry went to first grade the teacher would not tolerate her behavior, would put her desk outside the classroom and generally ignore her. After the principal told me that she needed to be spanked I finally went to the assistant superintendent about this kind of treatment. He made arrangements for the school psychologist to see her. She was allowed to stay in the classroom after that, but by the end of first grade she still could not read. After conferences with the second grade teacher, who was more sympathetic, we obtained a reading specialist for her and Terry began to make some progress, and eventually Ken and I decided to get her a horse and board it at a nearby farm owned by the Summerhill family. Ken was completely supportive, kind and patient with Terry and drove her out to the farm whenever she wanted to go riding– which was often. When nothing else seemed to calm her, or soothe her, the time she spent learning to ride and groom was deeply meaningful to her. Perhaps it saved her.

Exactly a year to the day after she graduated from high school, she left for Texas. She worked for a while and then called and asked us to cosign for a car for her. I refused and Ken agreed with me. But when he got on the phone with her he changed his mind and signed the loan. Shortly after that the car was repossessed or stolen, I never knew which. Terry was getting involved with drugs by that time, and her world was beginning to fall apart. She has been addicted on and off since then, creating dissention and anxiety in the family over our inability to help her.

I was furious. Margie was working, Jim was working for a computer company in Binghamton, New York and Ed was in college. Ken and I did not talk. Trying to argue with him about solutions seemed to make things worse. I went back to my standard problem solving recourse: run away from the problem.

I became even more determined to reclaim my own life. That year, 1982, I went to graduate school at the University of Indiana to get a masters degree in art therapy. I paid for it by working at Western Psychiatric Hospital as a nurse on weekends. After getting my degree, I worked at Western Psych for a short time, then went to work for Allegheny County Mental Health, a community mental health agency in Homestead, a suburb about an hour's drive from our house in Vandergrift, close to Pittsburgh.

In 1985, unable to quiet my anger, I rented an apartment close to the mental health center. My excuse was that it was too hard traveling back and forth every day to work, but the real reason was that I was still infuriated with Ken. The apartment was small, dark and above a saloon. I demanded that the landlord rent me another apartment that he owned on the street, but it was no good. After a few months I could not stand the loneliness. I would never in my life have considered getting a divorce. It was an impossible thought. Ken was too nice to divorce.

Ken came to visit often and wanted me to come back home. Finally I decided that my exasperation with him was not a good reason to continue to be stubborn. I thought that if I really tried to talk to Ken about what was happening, we could resolve my unhappy outbursts. We talked about being lonely when we were first married and made our own marriage vow that we would stay together. I told Ken that I didn't want to be angry any more, and that I wanted to come home. "We still love each other", I said to myself.

But love changes throughout the years. When we had children; our love moved toward them. When the children left it changed again; to a sense of companionship. "I think we can do more things together, and we can still be friends when we grow old." Ken just looked at me, and said "Thank you," and I gave him a long overdue hug and kiss.

"I'm sorry, Ken." I said. "I'm sorry I made you so sad." He put his arm around me as we went down the steps of my apartment. So I came home. I became more patient and we were more loving to each other. And life became more pleasant.

We decided to go to Florida after Christmas. Terry had been there for a year, and we had gone there once before, to search for her after not having had any communications from her for more than a month.

On January 27, 1986, our thirty-fifth wedding anniversary, Ken and I were in the Newark airport, a stop on our way to Florida to try to find Terry for the second time. We had not heard from her since December when she had sent me a Christmas present, a library book that was probably stolen. This was a symbol to me that something was seriously wrong. She had probably lost her job, and had no money. We knew that she had become part of the drug culture rampant in Florida in the 1970s and early 1980s, had convinced her the year before to go to drug rehab. She had been keeping in touch on a fairly regular basis since then until she dropped out of sight again and sent me the book.

We, or maybe just I, decided that we had to go to Florida and find out what was going on. We went by People's Express, an inexpensive airline whose flights went to Newark Airport in New Jersey before going on to a final destination. All of the televisions in the waiting area were tuned to a channel that was focused on the lift off of Challenger Space shuttle that was going up that morning. I watched as the astronauts, in their bulky space suits, held their helmets, smiling and waving to the crowds behind barriers, and filed onto the spacecraft.

The line was forming for the passengers on our flight as the countdown for the lift off began. I was entranced by the beautiful orange flames that shot out from the platform as the rocket slowly began to rise before it angled off into the atmosphere. I assumed all was going well because shuttle trips had become almost routine. I watched the smoke trailing the flames. The airport was suddenly quiet, as if everybody there was holding their breath. I looked at the nearest screen and saw that the smoke had changed from a stream to a widening cloud that gradually let out sparks, shades of orange and blue and black. The shuttle disappeared in the eerie chaotic mix.

"It's exploded," somebody whispered behind me. "Oh, my God! It's exploded!" became a lament repeated endlessly throughout the airport waiting room. Too shocked to think about what was happening, Ken and I silently got on the plane with the other passengers, all of us like robots.

I felt like this was our own tragic journey. We had Terry's address and telephone number so I called there and found out that none of the other three roommates had seen her for about a week. They gave us a phone number of an acquaintance who might have seen her but he denied knowing anything about her situation. The link led to more links until I finally talked to one who said they had seen her in a nearby park earlier that day.

We found Terry sitting on a bench, with Domino, her golden haired Afghan dog beside her on the ground. She may have been sleeping because she jumped up, tightened her hold on Domino's leash, her eyes shifting to look behind me. She made a move to run but I grabbed her arm and held on to her. Her clothes looked like they were scavenged from a barrel, they were so dirty, her usual pristine look further ravaged by tangled hair, no makeup, and skin that had faded from summer tan to dark yellow.

"It's me, Terry. Mom." I said as calmly as I could. My arm was shaking, my heart was beating wildly. The feeling of death after the shuttle disaster was still there.

She stared at me. "Mom?" She looked around, checked the landscape. "Where's Dad?"

"Right there across from us, on the bench." I pointed. She covered her face and said: "I don't want him to see me."

"It's OK, " I said. "I wanted to talk to you first. I need to find out what happened and what we need to do to help."

"No." she said and tried to pull away. I held her arm so tight that it must have hurt but it kept her there. "I'm not letting you go until you tell me what's going on." She gave me that defiant look that was her strength and her weakness. "Please, Terry, tell me."

She looked across at her Dad and perhaps could see the agony in his distancing himself from her pain. She kept watching him, sat on the ground and put her head on Domino's back. She didn't look at me for a long while.

"I forged my friend's name on one of his checks." Her voice was muted through the dog's soft fur. "He said he called the police and they were looking for me." She was terrified that the police were looking for her and had been wandering around, bunking with friends, afraid to go back to her apartment.

I wrapped my arms around her and held her close, refusing to release my hold. I told her that we had talked to all of her friends and none of them had mentioned police so maybe her friend had not called the police. "He did, I know he did. He said he would."

"OK" I said, after a long silence. "We're going to call the police and find out. You can't keep running, it will only get worse. We're here. We'll do whatever we need to do to help you." She started to cry, too tired to resist any longer.

She led me to a pay phone and I called. A pleasant voice informed me that there was no record of any call about her and asked to talk to her. After a few minutes she stopped crying. The police had never been notified and said that the bank would have notified them if they wanted her arrested. It was the bank's problem and if she would talk to them she could probably get it taken care of. She sat down on the grass, her hand still clinging to Domino's leash and started crying again. "I'm so tired," she said. "Could we go home?"

Ken watched me as I forced her to stay with me, but he stayed on that bench until we started to leave. I was angry with him, but I could only think of what had to be done, not how either of us was feeling. At the time I didn't understand how profoundly Terry's behavior had affected Ken.

When we returned home, I was unable to separate the tragedy of Terry from that of the explosion of the Challenger and had nightmares about it for a long time. I also was unable to reconcile Ken's inability to confront Terry. I felt that Ken had abandoned me when I needed him. But as time passed, I gradually began to realize that he was depressed. Unfortunately I was unable to indentify his behavior as depression until we started to see a psychologist a few years later, who was able to get him to talk about his feelings. She recommended that he see a psychiatrist, who then prescribed an antidepressant for him.

I found out from those sessions with the psychologist that Ken had always been afraid he would hurt someone if he got angry. I didn't understand that he had trouble making independent decisions, and that my determination to make necessary decisions gave him little room for participation. Luckily for me he was good with the children, listened to them, took them places, paid attention to them, and usually did whatever they asked him to. I loved him for those qualities. I think seeing Terry in such a state in Florida was too much for him to handle. He had spent a lifetime avoiding conflict and was unable to change in a crisis.

I forgave Ken for the betrayal I felt in Florida. The image that stayed with me was that of Ken, hunched over on a park bench, looking up at us with a mournful look, unable to make himself move. He was lost. When I thought of him in that moment, I reminded myself what it meant to be alone and frightened.

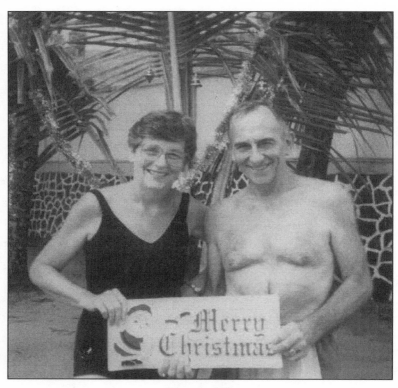

Anna and Ken
Indonesia December, 1987

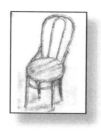

CHAPTER THREE

That same year, 1986, the United States Steel Corporation was looking for people to go to Indonesia for a two-year period and they asked Ken if he would be interested. When he told me about it I was excited, but he didn't say much, so I decided not to try to talk him into taking the job. However, I didn't object when our children Margie and Ed tried to convince him that he should take advantage of the opportunity to spend his last working years seeking a bit of adventure. Ken was 62 and I was 59, the timing was ripe.

Terry assured us that she would be all right and was going to stay in Florida. We kept in touch with her and hoped for the best. So, three months after we came home from that tragic trip to Florida, Ken took the job offer be a quality control met-allurgist in a new steel mill in Indonesia. The chance to travel, to visit new and exotic places was exciting to me. Margie and

Ed were hoping that we would go and they could spend some time there. Ken finally said that "Maybe it would be good."

On the day before leaving, I remember sitting on the carpet in our house in Vandergrift, where we had lived for twenty three years, having a wild crying episode. Ken had dropped a favorite sculpture, one that I had made ten years before. I thought it had broken, and the leaving time was close, so it was a relief to have a concrete reason for crying. Two large windows filled the room with light. The house was empty of furniture, but not bare. It was full of reflections from the trees and the sky, as my mind was full of reflections of our life there. I somehow had always thought of the Vandergrift house as belonging to my husband and the kids, but that day I could see which part was mine.

I was saying goodbye but was glad to be going far away from the emotional ties that had become a burden through the years. I wanted to leave my children to get on with their own lives. It seemed like time to break the family commitments that had kept me in place for so long. My sister Betty, who had moved back to Pittsburgh after retirement to be near me, was now in an assisted living facility and almost blind. And my youngest sister Margie, a Sister of St. Joseph nun, was still in the convent but lived independently in her own apartment near our house.

I knew there was not much I could do for them at this point. I wanted to leave the worries, the caring for others that I had done for so long, all the accumulated emotional ties. I hoped that I would be able to find out if I could live with myself when I didn't feel obliged to do anything for anybody else.

I wanted to do the things I had always planned to do when I retired. I had kept journals since my teens and wanted to learn more about writing and do more painting.

As we were driving to the airport Ken pointed out a rainbow bowing across the sky. No wonder people attribute magical things to rainbows. They are so beautiful. The colors were brilliant for a few seconds and then gradually became soft and wispy, then drifted away. I had seen few rainbows in my lifetime and it was one of those moments of pure joy that have stayed with me all my life. Now I understand why people look for omens. This felt like one; it somehow banished the fear I had about going half way around the world to spend two years away from all that was familiar.

We flew north, across parts of Canada, then west over Alaska, the colors changing from green to darker green to browns and blacks. The clouds drifted along, pure white shadowed to grey at times. Sometimes I could see a filmy layer of earth below, as over western Canada, some mountain tops jutting up through the clouds. After about twenty hours in the air and a night in an outrageously luxurious hotel in Singapore, (where, for some unknown reason, all the expatriates had to register with some bureaucracy before being allowed to enter Indonesia), we finally arrived at our new home in Cilegon, a rural town in Indonesia three hours drive from Jakarta, the capitol of Indonesia, where the steel mill had recently been built.

Our new house was a modern design, with window walls looking out into gardens on every side and trees in front with branches that twisted at odd angles from a round knobs. I was enthralled by the naturally lighted space.

It took some weeks before everything became more than impressions that shone through a hazy layer of sunshine. I felt suspended in some other world, one like my childhood where everything was done in a simple way. Clothes were washed by hand, spread out on the floor and scrubbed with a brush; the men carried dirt in small pails for filling holes in the yard, resulting from the theft of flowering bushes; the tile floors were washed on hands and knees, using old, soft cloths. The women carried their babies in a cloth wrapped close to the mother's side and we seldom heard a baby cry.

Most of the Indonesian people that we came to know well were working for us. They were small and quiet and very industrious, always polite. After getting to know them they became friendly and more vocal and tried to help us with their language. They seldom wore bright colors and yet it was obvious that they loved color; they would choose the bright-est colors when shopping for anything other than clothing. It was almost as if the Indonesians needed to be unobtrusive. The Indonesians did things so quietly and beautifully I felt like a big bumpkin at times. At first it was puzzling that they seemed to appreciate beauty in so many ways and did not see anything ugly in the cluttered environment. There were small mountains of plastic bags and other non-biodegradable litter surrounding the local villages. The Indonesians didn't seem to notice it pile up or allow it to intrude on their sense of order.

I finally decided that they were long accustomed to biodegradable waste, and that maybe they assumed that all the plastic would just eventually disappear back into the rainforest.

I floated through Indonesia selfishly, enjoying the scenery, the exotic experience of everything. Or Indonesia wandered through me. I saw, I reflected, I lived free of emotional encumbrances, other than momentary ones. What a gift it was! It seemed to be all light.

Now, when life is harder in a different way and so much has changed, I think often of the wild, white surf waves at Carita beach that laughingly pounded into the fine, white sand. I think of the placid waves at Merak, the drooping palms, the burning beach that I sampled only occasionally when I stepped out from under the protection of the umbrella. I think of the pleasant young men teaching Batik who called me "Ibu", grandmother, and treated me with such teasing respect. There was deep satisfaction in the languid life. I had no insecurities and few anxieties. I was floating on a wave of serenity that made me feel quiet and introspective; carried along by the warmth and the breeze.

We spent two years suspended in that other world. For the first time in my life I didn't worry what others thought of me. I felt happy with myself. I think Ken was happy, too. He went to the mill every day in the "combie", the name given to the van with passenger seats that two Western families shared. Ken was content with the work, found it interesting, and became friendly with the men he traveled with to work. He worked closely with the Chinese working at the mill, teaching them how to monitor the quality of the steel and how to write reports, and formed a real friendship with a colleague, a Dutch metallurgist, who kept in touch with Ken for years after we returned home.

I had requested work before we left home, and was given the job of teaching school to American children, and also was the nurse on call for health issues. The house was run by Yoyo, our house girl; the car was taken care of by Yudia, our driver, all paid for by US Steel. I taught in the mornings and had time to spend most afternoons at the beach. Ken was not interested in going to the beach. Instead, we explored Jakarta and Bali and the islands that make up Indonesia, sometimes with the other couples, most times just the two of us. Ken was content at home, too. For Ken, the change in lifestyle was just as important, or maybe more so. The pressure of the worries at home were far away. We had a lot of good times together and became closer.

Those were good years for us. I was a world away from the problems I had been struggling with. I felt free, made friends, realized the value of my nursing and observation skills. Most importantly, I was able to secure help for Ken when he had what seemed to be an allergy on his face. We did not have an American doctor there. The only doctor was French and he did not seem interested. I reported to our project manager that I was not satisfied with their diagnosis, and they had Ken sent to Singapore for treatment. A nurse went with him, and I went along and spent two lovely weeks in Singapore while he was being treated for shingles.

Ken was due to retire when he was sixty five, but his birthday occurred when we were in Indonesia, so he was able to extend his retirement. It was all right at first. We'd rented our house in Vandergrift to a young family when we left for Indonesia and they offered to buy the house when we returned. After two years of rest and relaxation, and the precious sense of re-connecting to the world, I refused to move back to Vandergrift. So in 1988 we sold the house.

I had never been satisfied with living in a small town and now I wanted to live in the city so I could take advantage of the various art classes available, in addition to better job choices. I never felt accepted in Vandergrift, either, perhaps because I worked and did not socialize with many other people. Two women that I had become friends with had moved out of town by the time we returned. Ken would have stayed there and retired, but I was unwilling to do so.

We rented an apartment in a suburb of Pittsburgh, close to the city. Terry was now in a drug rehab center nearby, so we were able to see her fairly often. Ken was asked to delay his retirement for a year and work at the nearby Irvin Mill, part of the U.S. Steel Corporation, to help in the metallurgy department. He was pleased with the offer and that he could earn money for one more year.

The following year, 1989, Ken officially retired and we moved to Philadelphia. At that time my son-in-law Edwin was a woodworker with a small business, and Ken had been a hobbyist in wood working for many years. I thought we were going to Philadelphia to help Edwin, Margie's husband, and for Ken to apprentice him to learn about woodworking. We went through our usual muddled way of making this decision. I thought he wanted to go and he thought he was going because I wanted to go.

I didn't pay a lot of attention to Ken at first. I took a Saturday morning class in jewelry making class at Temple University in Philadelphia, where I learned how to photograph my work, how to display it, and how to sell it. I loved the class, and learned a lot in that one semester. I sold several large bracelets in Philadelphia, and was able to continue creating and selling.

Eventually I realized that Ken did nothing but sit and read or watch television when he came home from working with Edwin, and didn't talk except to say how tired he was. With no small amount of guilt, I began to feel I'd forced him into something he didn't want. Maybe he just wanted to stay in Vandergrift, which was so much like the small town of Mercer, where he grew up.

About eight months later we decided to move back to Pittsburgh. In 1990, we bought a cottage in Edgewood, a small leafy suburb near where we had rented an apartment the year before. The house needed a lot of work, but we didn't think that was a problem. I assumed that Ken had some new woodworking skills from working with Edwin, and I thought he might be happier; he would have a project to work on. It was one decision we both could agree on.

But it turned out to be too much physical work for him, and he had a lot of anxiety.

Ken started to replace the floor boards on the front porch, but got frustrated and gave up after fixing a few of the worst ones. He finally left the remainder of the work to the remodelers. He tried to build a stone wall along the side of the house, and spent long months working away at it for short spells.

At first, I thought he missed the kids, that he was experiencing "empty nest" syndrome. I felt bad about all the confusion in our move to Philadelphia, but to me it offered a fruitful promise similar to our interlude in Indonesia. Looking back, Ken probably did not want to go to Indonesia either, but he was active and happy there once he got settled. Unfortunately the time in Philadelphia did not work out that way.

So, I couldn't help much with the renovation, and Ken couldn't manage it. Ken was always a physically active person (unlike me) and loved sports. All of the 25 years we lived in Vandergrift he walked to work, played tennis, and jogged. He prided himself on being in shape and always looked sharp and took care of his clothes. He was physically graceful – a quality that he has never lost, even now. But this time he didn't have the energy to force himself to do the work. Fortunately, this time I was paying attention and was able to respond.

I went back to work at the community mental health center and used the money to pay for a contractor to finish the job. The house became comfortable and had a warm bright feeling. We fixed up the basement with an extra bedroom and bathroom, and added a wood workshop for Ken. Ken volunteered for the Eastern Area for the Aging in Pittsburgh. After a few months they offered him a job and he soon was earning some money there by shopping for groceries and delivering them to elderly people. Everybody at the office liked him, and he was happy being a helper to people in need and became much livelier than he had been.

I liked our new life in Edgewood too. The streets were tree lined, the houses were well taken care of and the neighbors were friendly. I joined a poetry workshop at Carlow University in Pittsburgh called Mad Women in the Attic. This was a weekly workshop for community women led by poet Patricia Dobler, Director of the Creative Writing program at Carlow. Pat was a skilled poet and an inspired teacher. I think one of the reasons the workshop was so transformative was that she collected the student writing and published an annual volume of our work. As her student in the workshop, I felt that my voice was heard and that our work was valued. This really helped me to have the confidence to begin writing about my life.

Most of the poems I wrote in the workshop were about my childhood and my family. When Pat was sick, a substitute teacher suggested that I should transpose the poems I had been writing in class into prose, because it seemed obvious to him that I wanted to tell the story of my family. This was a thrilling idea to me, and was the beginning of my writing more intentionally about myself.

In Edgewood we were close to our daughter Terry, who by this time was working off and on for her boyfriend, a recovered addict who was immensely patient with her and helped her. We had fairly separate lives and I did not ask too many questions – a strategy I have employed throughout my life when I was uncertain of the answers. I remember some of the things that happened, but I don't want to write about it because it is too painful for me to remember. I suppose I have blocked them out. It's like going through a relentless storm – I didn't think, I just went through it.

After the time in Florida, I hoped for the best but was always cautious about what I expected. From all those years of working in mental health I knew the odds were not in favor of someone being able to heal from their addictions, but as a mother I clung to some kind of hope.

One day in 1998, when Ken was jogging, he had mild chest pain, not enough for him to tell me at the time. When it happened a second time, he told me. I took him to see a doctor immediately. An angioplasty showed that although some of the blood vessels close to the heart were entirely closed, he had not suffered any damage to the heart muscle. The angioplasty surgery was botched the first time. The doctor was inexperienced and could not get the catheter into all of the arteries and it had to be done again two days later. When Ken could talk, he was explosive and angry, and demanded something for the pain. I was surprised and a bit pleased at this new side of him.

For the next two years we paid little attention to his heart, muddling along trying to resolve our accumulating problems with Ken's depression. We allowed Terry to live at home again but her ongoing addiction, erratic behavior, and constant mood swings, added to my frustration. I tried to keep from getting despondent.

Ken and I went to a therapy group for families of addicts at Western Psychiatric Institute in Pittsburgh. We felt desperate and I knew that I needed help. The psychologist who facilitated the group was skilled and compassionate. When the group sessions were over, I asked Sally if we could have some private sessions with her and she agreed. Sally helped Ken and I to resolve some of our problems with Terry and with each other. Ken was less silent and I made fewer angry remarks; we were gradually able to

communicate a bit better. Sally sent Ken to a psychiatrist who prescribed an antidepressant, which seemed to gradually cheer him
up.

In early 2000 Ken sliced off part of his thumb when he
was using the table saw in his basement wood shop. Not without feeling guilty now, I remember hurriedly wrapping a tour-
niquet around his thumb while reminding him how often I had
asked him not to use the saw in the evening because his judgment
declined at that time of day. Looking back, I see that impaired
judgment is one of the early symptoms of dementia, but at the
time I knew next to nothing about the disease or that there was
the remotest possibility of his having it. I see now the depression and inertia after Ken's first heart attack were among the
unidentified symptoms of cognitive impairment from a dementia that I did not recognize. I was feeling my way in the dark, just
as I had done with Terry when I was trying to understand what
was happening to her.

I drove Ken to the nearby hospital and Terry came with us.
We arrived around midnight and Ken was immediately rushed
into surgery. He lost part of his thumb, below the nail. Terry was
very upset, and we talked about what she was feeling guilty about.
She said she was afraid it happened because she'd been arguing
with him, but wouldn't say anymore. She was in crisis again. She
was trying to stay clean, but it was a terrible struggle. I felt sadder
for her than I did for Ken. Bad as it was for him, he still would
have the use of his hand.

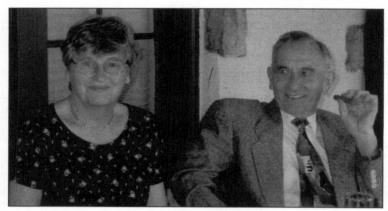

Anna and Ken
Pittsburgh June, 1998

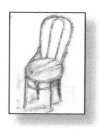

CHAPTER FOUR

In 2001, early on a dreary November morning, the horrific events of September 11th still fresh and unthinkable, I found Ken slumped in his favorite chair in the living room. Only his eyes moved, a slow shift of his pupils to meet mine. The early morning sun struggled to illuminate his face but only reached the green velour of the chair, making his face even more shadowed and grey.

"Ken, what's wrong?" I asked, leaning over him and touching his wrist to find a pulse.

His voice just a whisper. "I took a pill."

"What kind of pill?"

His eyes shifted again. "I don't know."

"Mom! What's wrong with Dad?" Terry's voice rose to a screech "Call 911!"

"Get the car started," I said, my response almost automatic, "I'll call the doctor and tell him we are going to the emergency room. It will be faster. An ambulance will take longer. You get the car started. " She grabbed her car keys and rushed out to the driveway. Thinking about the car calmed her; driving is a thing she could do well. There was little traffic on the expressway to the hospital, so it must have just after before six in the morning. I remember the trees on the hillside were almost black, and most of the leaves were gone. I saw death in every dark branch.

When we arrived at the emergency room at the University of Pittsburgh Medical Center (UPMC) ten minutes later, Ken was immediately carried off for testing while I gave the critical information to the nurse. As I sat waiting in the emergency room for information, I remembered the image just a short while before of Ken in the chair, and the feeble winter sun struggling to reach Ken's face as if his life depended on it. At the time, I could only think of what I knew was a heart attack.

After an hour or so a nurse informed us that Ken was stable but needed to be kept in the hospital until further decisions were made. By that time Terry was extremely anxious, pacing the hallway and constantly asking the nurse for more information.

"Terry," I said, "Why don't you go home." She went, reluctantly, and I promised to call her if anything changed and when I needed a ride home.

Another hour passed before I was able to go to Ken's room. He opened his eyes, raised his hand slightly when I came in. His face felt cold when I kissed him, but he tried a smile before he closed his eyes again.

Several young doctors were huddled in the hall talking to each other. I asked to speak to the cardiologist and one of them told me they were his assistants. I asked them to tell me what was happening but they were unable to say much, either because they didn't know or were not senior enough to be permitted to give out much information. One of them mentioned that open-heart surgery was always a possibility and Ken would need to make that decision.

"They don't know," I thought. Ken's brother had a double bypass open heart surgery and he suffered severe dementia as a consequence - maybe due to even more loss of blood to the brain during surgery. The same thing happened to the husband of one of my friends, and she consequently spent all of her time staying at home to care for him, much as my friend Alice wrote about in her heartbreaking letter at the beginning of this book. They both became increasingly isolated; they rarely saw their friends like me. I was also aware of the problems in dealing with dementia through my experience at Western Psychiatric Institute, a division of the hospital Ken was in now. I didn't have much influence in the situation, but I knew enough about how the system worked to know that I could be a knowledgeable advocate.

"I would like to talk to the cardiologist, please," I said. After some discussion the cardiology residents agreed to ask the attending cardiologist to come and talk to me. He arrived a short time later, minus the white coat, black hair disheveled, and reached out to shake my hand.

"I am Dr. Condales, the cardiologist," he said as he lightly touched my shoulder to guide me into Ken's room. "Open heart surgery is an option, but I don't think it is the best choice for you." He was speaking to Ken, but looking at me as he said it. "He may not have enough good heart muscle left to do that." He then further explained that Ken would be in the hospital for a few more days while he and his team considered the best alternative for him to heal and to allow his heart to function at the best possible level.

Ken came home after a few days with a list of medications, and a strong suggestion that he should have cardiac rehabilitation. The cardiologist had recommended an experimental treatment, called Enhanced External Counterpulsation (EECP), referred to by the staff as the "hydraulic pants". Every day for six weeks Ken would go to the University of Pittsburgh Medical Center and put on a pair of pressure pants similar to the ones astronauts wore. The treatment involved a series of six specialized inflatable blood pressure cuffs that pumped blood from the legs back to the heart. The cuffs, three on each leg, were synchronized by a cardiac monitor that moves the blood in rhythm to the heart. The theory behind this was that as it pushed blood back toward the heart, (as the body muscles would if a person was running, for example) the patient would start to form new blood vessels that would compensate for those that were damaged. For Ken, it worked.

After the first series of treatment he was able to go back to driving and to his job grocery shopping part-time for the Eastern Area for the Aging.

The treatment was an advantage for me as well. Since I had to drive Ken to the hospital and stay for more than an hour each day, I spent that time working on the autobiographical stories that I had begun writing years before with the Mad Women in the Attic writing workshop.

At that point my thoughts were unclear. I couldn't write about what was happening now, I didn't want to think about the future. It was too close, unpredictable, and terrifying. I couldn't think about Ken because even after all these years together, I didn't really know much about his inner life. As I have said before, we never were good at explaining ourselves to each other. So I decided that I could write toward a new understanding of my childhood.

In those hours of waiting for Ken I began rereading the poems I had written years earlier, and reading through journals from my earlier life. I found a comfortable chair in the corner of the hospital hallway, and began to write the story of my life. This was the beginning of developing a clear artistic goal for my late years, which has sustained me through the writing of this memoir. The writing I started in the hospital later became "My Charles Street", a memoir about my immigrant parents and trying to understand the world of my lonely childhood during the depression of the 1930s in Pittsburgh.

By 2002, a year after the heart attack, the dementia was becoming more obvious, and our home became a battleground filled with resentment, confusion and depression for all concerned. When a person survives an illness you breathe a sigh of relief. But the process of recovery from severe stroke or massive heart attack can be filled with pitfalls, most of them unexpected and most of them leaving the caretaker completely in the dark about what is happening to that person. It certainly was a challenge to understand what was happening to me.

Terry had been going to Narcotic Anonymous meetings and working when she could. But she still had addiction problems. I knew what was happening to her, but did not yet have the energy or will to face it. Ferociously cleaning the house diverted some of the worry energy, but I felt guilty and incompetent. When I can't cope with anything else, I can always cope with sorting through dirt and disorder. Cleaning was my job as a child, and it still calms me down and helps to re-order my inner life.

Ken was becoming more lethargic. He was not sleeping regularly, and did not have energy for ordinary things. He just sat in his chair all day unless I prodded him to do something. He needed much more of my help than he had in the past. But even then, I was not relating his depression to his heart condition. I still had not put the pieces together.

Managing our money was becoming a problem. Throughout our married life, Ken never wanted me to make decisions about how to spend it. He spent it the way he wanted to and there was none left to do what I wanted. I felt that I was a coward and was afraid of fighting with him because there had been too many fights in our raucous Irish family. When I was insistent with Ken, intent on telling him what I wanted or felt that I needed, this led to arguments. Ken's way of dealing with emotions or negativity was to sulk, refuse to talk about the issue, or to answer my questions. This behavior drove me to fury. The sequence was that I would get really frustrated, then cry. He wouldn't talk. Sometimes we would drift back to talking again, but nothing was resolved because we did not communicate about whatever real issues were causing conflict.

One day, during this period of time, I was paying the bills. Ken was sitting beside me, sulking. He looked at me and said: "Do you want me to do anything?"

"Why don't you do something instead of asking me to make the decisions?"

I asked him.

"I'm just the one who has to follow orders of the one in charge," he said.

For a change, I was speechless. He was telling me in the words that he knew that something different was happening and that he was aware of it. He couldn't do a lot of the things he had done before; he was forgetting much more than old age would account for. He had always been reluctant to make decisions, but now he seemed unable to make them, constantly asking questions about whatever we were doing or about to do. Always "Do you want to?", never "I want" or "I will."

Little things bothered him. He became impatient easily, and talked even less than he did before. He did admit that it was hard to get up in the morning, but he didn't seem to want to do anything, and sulked all day. When that happened, we were often angry with each other.

Almost every day when Ken got home from his grocery shopping job there were new dents on the car. The front door on the passenger side had been bashed up and the paint was scraped. When the front hood became crinkled and wouldn't close, I realized that he was having accidents and could one day have a serious one. I tried to get him to stop driving, which meant leaving his job. I was reluctant to do that, but finally had no choice and he sadly agreed. What was happening to Ken was not simply aging.

Even though at this point we had not been to a doctor to assess Ken's mental status, it finally occurred to me that I needed to find out more about dementia. Through my work as a nurse in psychiatry, I was familiar with the end results of severe dementia but knew little about early symptoms and how to manage those to keep them from becoming completely debilitating. The doctors took good care of Ken's physical problems but never mentioned the possibility of changes to the brain. I never heard the word "dementia" used by any doctor, nor did any of them suggest support groups after Ken finished the physical therapy.

Although now, in 2014, it is a word used commonly by the medical profession and the general public, it is often associated with weary caretakers and a sense of dread, rather than as a diagnosis with treatment options. It is hard to distinguish the difference between normal mental changes that can occur with aging, and the changes from dementia.

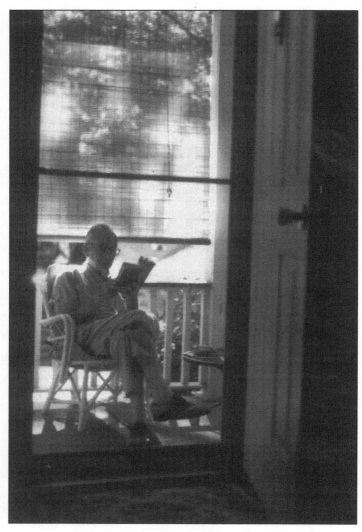

Ken reading on the porch
Pittsburgh July, 2002

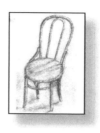

CHAPTER FIVE

By 2003, two years after Ken's heart attack, I was the one who was depressed. I cried more, not just tears discreetly shed, but loud crying jags that came out of nowhere. I had nightmares, was apprehensive and pessimistic, guilty, and believed that that nobody could help me. It's easy enough to say 'don't feel guilty', but in my life the guilt always stays there, a deep, grabbing, sudden smothering of anxiety that leads to anger and immobility.

Terry had relapsed. She had been doing cocaine and heroin again and Ken had been giving her money, believing whatever lie she said about what she was going to do with it. I knew she was using the money to buy drugs and I felt completely outraged. She balked and would not talk to me when I screamed at her. Not the most effective thing to do, but I thought there was no other way to get her to hear me. I decided that something had to change and that it was up to me to make the change. I decided not to care any more what Ken said or did or wanted to do about her.

I felt betrayed by Ken, even though I suspected that I must be half the problem. I could not think seriously about leaving, but it was more and more clear that something was wrong with Ken's mind. He was far from the kind, pleasant man that he had been before all of this began to happen. We had both been guilty of enabling Terry initially, but since his heart attack he could not refuse her anything. He gave her money, lent her our car and would not see what was happening. Terry needed to leave. The path we were on was doing nothing but harm.

I confronted Terry one day after I had seen Ken handing her the keys to our car. I grabbed the keys and told her that I would not fight about her with Ken any more and that I could not handle both of them. I reminded her that we had tried to help her when she came home after nine years in Florida. Our kind of help was ineffectual, and she needed professional help again. I had no choice except to tell her that she had to leave. I thought she would lock me out of our house as she had done a previous time when I asked her to go. But she went down to her basement room, gathered up some clothes and stormed out of the house. A week or so later I heard from one of her friends she was in a treatment center; the best thing for her at that time.

One of the things I felt very strongly about as a mother was that children should not be blindly obedient, that they should be able to make decisions themselves; that they should grow up and be independent people. Had I caused this?

I was haunted by a story from when our daughter Margie was six years old and just starting Catholic school. In 1958 there was a tragic fire at a Catholic School in Chicago. The most horrifying thing to me was that one of the school nuns had told her class to sit at their desks and pray, and the whole obedient class of children died from smoke inhalation. Ninety two children died. I wonder now if this incident and the powerful effect it had on my was part of the reason for my allowing more freedom than was good and safe for our children?

A few days after Terry left, I spent some time down in the basement looking at some of my old paintings that were stacked up in Ken's wood shop. One was a large portrait of myself that I had painted in 1970, the year Margie graduated from high school. In this painting I was standing framed in a doorway alone, with nothing on either side of me except space. I remember I had worked on it for weeks. In one of my darkest moments I remember talking to the painting, saying "I want to quit, I want to leave, but I can't!"

I did not look at it again for a more than a year. At that time, in 1970, I thought Ken hated me. I was having nightmares about climbing familiar streets from my childhood that were ever higher and steeper, but never ended. I dreamt about trying to get out of a house with many rooms and no doors, again familiar dream images. I felt boxed in and couldn't find a way out. I realize now that my own painting showed me my feelings and my state of mind, but I couldn't do anything about it at that time.

Whenever I want to really think about myself, I have continued to look at that painting and remember that day I spent back in 1970 in the basement wondering what to do with my life and railing against the message my own artwork was communicating to me; a reminder of an unhappiness that I did not want to repeat.

Twenty three years later in 2003, I pulled that old painting out into the light and looked at my posture, my unhappy face, my dreary clothing, and remembered another painting that I had done even earlier, years before in the early 1960s when the children were young. Nursing jobs were hard to get at that time and I was feeling that I wanted something more in life. That time I did a painting of a black lantern with a bright flame. I remembered the tears splashing over my arm and the brush as I slashed in the orange and yellow fire until it was barely contained in the lantern. By the time I finished that painting I was clearly looking at my anger, my resentment, my anxiety - none of which I could articulate.

That painting expressed my feelings. And the clarity of it helped me, at the time, to develop a plan. I had become friends with a married couple across our back alley. Bill, the husband, was Dean of the night school at Penn State in New Kensington, a town about ten miles away from Vandergrift where we were living in 1977. He was a sensitive friend who recognized my depression and encouraged me to attend classes. When I agreed, he immediately suggested a list of the classes and found a student who was taking classes on the same nights as I was who I could ride with. I started with the study of chemistry. Learning was exciting, as it had always been for me, and I kept right on going.

The following year, 1978, I registered at Seton Hill College in Greensburg, Pennsylvania, a nearby small liberal arts school. I asked for financial help from the school and was offered the job of nurse in their health center for a twenty-four hour stretch on the weekends during each term. I attended classes one or two days a week for three years under this arrangement, and was given a financial grant for my final year of college. I earned a bachelors degree in art, and several years later I took classes at the Indiana University of Pennsylvania, graduating with a masters degree in art therapy in 1984.

Painting has always helped me see my emotional life more clearly. Remembering those paintings from earlier years helped me to realize that I was depressed again, and had to do something to save my mental and emotional life. These memories, and the advice from our children, finally convinced me to get help.

Ken and I both went back to see the psychologist from Western Psychiatric hospital who had helped us before. She was able to help me see that I needed to be more actively helpful in boosting Ken's self esteem. She also helped me to realize that a lot of the problems I had were because of my own chaotic childhood which didn't teach me to sort out my feelings, nor to make affirmative decisions based on what I needed.

So I began to be nicer to Ken and consciously tried to quit complaining about my own problems. Well, I didn't quit completely, but I did better. Sally, the psychologist, helped me to realize that I had always been afraid of losing control of my life, and that this fear had been controlling me.

We were advised not to let Terry live at home again. Ken and I were at odds about that, insisting that there was no way we could keep her out. I finally bought some new doorknobs with locks and told him we had to change the locks on both the front and back doors of the house.

The next day I came home from shopping and found a huge hole in the front door. Ken was kneeling in front of it with a doorknob and a screwdriver in his hand. When I asked Ken what he was doing his response was: "Well, you told me to change the locks!" At that point I remembered Sally's words, and realized that it was not fear of losing control of my life, I had by now completely lost control of my life.

My research on dementia helped me to understand that Ken had been suffering from depression; and that many people with dementia are caught in a cycle of depression, which results in less and less motivation to continue their usual activities and contributes to a lack of interest in the world around them. Finally realizing that Ken was depressed helped me to look at my own feelings and to get rid of some of the guilty feelings that I had been focusing on.

Our children, Jim, Margie and Ed, were offering to help us, giving advice, urging us to move near them, but I wasn't listening, and Ken did not know what was going on. I finally accepted that I had to make the decision to accept the help that our children were offering me. I resolved not to ever enable Terry again. She would have to learn to live her own life, the only way to give me room to live mine. I needed her to play a minor role in our lives the way that our other children did. My need to focus on Ken was also the major part of my decision to move away from our house in Pittsburgh and everything that was familiar to me.

Our son and daughter, Ed and Margie, had been offering us to live with one of them. Ed had an apartment in his house in New York and Margie and her husband Edwin had moved into a larger house in Philadelphia. Our son Jim and daughter-in-law Cindy also said we could move in with them, but living with them in an isolated house on a mountain top near Pittsburgh, would not have helped the depression that had descended on us. I needed to be in a city with public transportation, opportunities for classes and other cultural opportunities, and easy access to good health care.

In 2004, it seemed that Ed's offer of a second floor apartment in Queens, New York would be the best alternative. We would pay rent and have our own apartment. Ed and our daughter in law, Merin, and our grandchildren Jack and Sadie would live on the first floor and we would live in the apartment above. But it would turn out that the move to Queens was as lonely as the rural house of Jim's would have been.

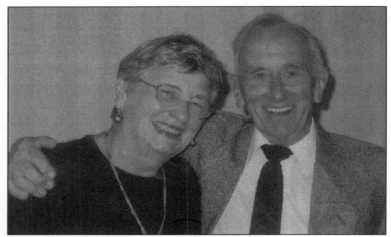

Anna and Ken
Pittsburgh March, 2003

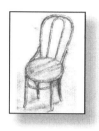

CHAPTER SIX

It was late summer of 2004 as we prepared to move to Ed's house in Ridgewood, Queens from Pittsburgh, where we had lived for fourteen years. The leaves on the trees still wore their summer green and whispered to each other. That was the sound I would miss more than any other when we moved.

The cottage house in Pittsburgh was small, one story, and Ken and I changed it in many ways. We had added a new porch, more windows, enlarged the kitchen and renovated the basement by adding a bathroom and a new furnace. The improvements, and the fact that the Edgewood section of Pittsburgh was a well-governed borough, meant that we had no trouble selling it.

The house that I grew up in during the 1930s was an attachment of a different sort: it was our family's house, not mine. That was a brick row house on Charles Street on the

North Side of Pittsburgh. To my childhood mind, the street and the house were all one. It was an attachment to a memory, a symbol of all the things that I did not understand about my life.

I think I grew up wondering "why". Why was our family different from the other families on the street? What were their houses like? Why weren't we allowed into their houses? We were warned not to talk to the neighbors. Why did we have to go a mile to a Catholic school when the public school was just around the corner? Why did our mother and father fight? Why did my brothers and sisters fight? Why did our father drink so much and stay away from home for such long times? Why was I always looking for corners to hide in? Why was there so much chaos? Some smart psychologist answered that for me about forty years later with her quote from a book about alcoholism: Children of alcoholics don't know what normal behavior is. They have to guess. Maybe I married Ken because he kept me guessing - and still does; a life long habit that may be tied to my upbringing.

My mother's house and our rigid Catholic practice were also symbolic of other qualities that I was not aware of until I had my own family: the need for conflict resolution, an unheard of term then, but definitely lacking in our family; caring, displayed by my mother in her constant acceptance of my father's return home after drinking bouts. I unknowingly absorbed some of the qualities that are part of the religion and were part of my life at home: compassion for those who seem dishonorable, wrong, sick or abandoned.

I had always thought that I would never get attached to merely a house. When I was growing up in my mother's house on Charles Street nothing was "my own." The Edgewood house was "my own." And then I lost it.

If I had not been so depressed and unable to make any other decision I would have stayed there. But the depression was taking over my whole life and I had to make a change. Sally, our intrepid psychologist, could have advised me, but I did not think to ask her. After I told Terry that we were leaving, she completely rebelled and dove into heavy drug usage again.

In Edgewood, I had always invited my two sisters, Betty and Margie, to our house for breakfast on Sunday mornings after they went to mass at the Catholic church. I enjoyed making breakfast and a weekly social ritual with my sisters. I was writing in the Mad Women in the Attic workshop at the time, and some of those poems were about my childhood. I remember reading them aloud to my sisters; their frequent comment: "I don't remember that! You must have grown up in a different family." But we were never able to explain what was different; they were as unable to talk about their feelings and their experience as I was. The closest we came to verbalizing real affection with each other was when I told them that we were moving. They both expressed how much they would miss me and the Sunday breakfasts. I hate to say it, but I was surprised.

It was only when I found out later that my sister Margie had been drinking all of her adult life and was a secret alcoholic, that I realized how much our Sunday meetings meant to her. She had a good mask. She functioned well as principal of a Catholic elementary school and hid her drinking from almost everybody in her life. Betty had a beginning cancer at that time and she kept that a secret, too. I realize now that I had my own mask when I was with them, too. I didn't tell them about Terry's problems, or my problems, because I was afraid that they would be shocked and disapproving. I didn't tell them about Ken's developing dementia, partly because I'm not sure I recognized it myself. I didn't tell them about the dementia until a short time before we decided to move east to live with our children.

Our son, Jim, was working near Pittsburgh at the time and came often after work and helped with all of the tribulations of moving to another city. He knew what we were going through because he had stayed with us for about six months when IBM closed the plant in New York where he worked several years before, and he had lived with us in Edgewood for the months it took to find a job in Pittsburgh, buy a house, and move his family.

Our house closing was scheduled for late September 2004. In the middle of that month Ken's brother John had a stroke. John was hospitalized in Pittsburgh, then sent to a stroke rehabilitation center nearby. John's home was about sixty miles north of where we lived, so I asked my sister in law, Annie, to stay with us while John was in the hospital and rehab. I cleared out a bedroom and she made it her home for the two weeks we were preparing to move.

Annie would come home from the hospital about nine o'clock every evening, and we would sit in our kitchen for hours, drinking tea and talking. We had become friends through the years of family gatherings, many of which I found boring. Discussions seemed to be completely related to babies, children, and neighbors, but Annie had always been ready to ask how things were going with me. This time when she asked, I told her everything: about Terry's problems, Ken's attitude, my worries about his mind, my sisters Betty and Margie's grief and some anger at my leaving them, even our shortage of money for the closing of the house sale. I listened to her worries about her husband John, the hospital and how she would care for him after he returned home. Annie listened more than she talked. Her attention and concern, during those evenings, didn't erase my anxieties, but did make them more bearable. Annie was the one person who helped me through the last few weeks of depression, anxiety and loneliness before we finally said goodbye to our life and made the move.

As I look back at that time now, I realize that Ken was not officially diagnosed with dementia until 2012. All of the eight years in between, I was acting on my own knowledge, my observations of his mother, his four brothers and one sister, all of whom were diagnosed with Alzheimer's disease. I had seen Alzheimer's up close when I worked at Western Psychiatric Hospital and consequently never believed that Ken's family members suffered from it. Four of his five siblings had a heart attack or a stroke before the symptoms appeared, and none of them had the sort of mood changes or severe language disability that was more typical of Alzheimer's.

In the 1960s, when Ken's mother Lucille was diagnosed with Alzheimer's, most cases of dementia were give that label. In retrospect, I think her symptoms were similar to the ones

Ken has now: loss of short-term memory, confusion, and agitation. She too could have had Vascular Dementia.

As long as I knew Lucille, she had some obsessive behaviors. She cleaned the house incessantly, and ironed everything, even the underwear. I thought it was because she had six children's worth of work to do, and was a lifelong housewife who took care of everything. When Lucille began to show signs of Alzheimer's, Ken's father, Walter, thought that it would help Lucille if they moved to a smaller, more convenient house. But after they moved, she wandered. Walter was there with her, but he was not in the habit of paying attention to her. He worked in the garden, and spent devoted hours listening to the baseball games on the radio, while Lucille was left to herself. She did not recognize where she was, and would drift off down the road, looking for her beloved old home on Beaver Street in Mercer, the town where Ken grew up.

During that time I remember Lucille sitting on a kitchen chair, her hands folded primly in her lap, her feet together, as if she were a debutant waiting to be asked to dance. It was a family gathering and some of her other relatives were visiting. Everyone decided to have their lunch outside in the yard of her little house. They tried to talk to her, but she looked at them vaguely and did not reply. They soon gave up and chattered among themselves. I think of this often when I see Ken sitting in a daze now at the dinner table, not able to understand or contribute to the conversation, and wonder what Lucille was feeling. Luckily Ken never wandered as his mother did. Maybe that was because I tried to pay attention, to stay with him, and to help him adjust to new conditions.

Ken had always been my source of help to keep the lonely demons away. We didn't talk a lot at times but we each knew that the other was always there. The dementia was taking him to another world in his mind and during this period of decline he became a stranger. He had reluctantly left his grocery shopping job with Pittsburgh Area for the Aging earlier in the summer. He had reached a point where he was sometimes confused about what to do and I thought he was having a hard time remembering where to go. I took over the driving until we sold the car, one of the last things I did before we left Pittsburgh the last time. I felt sure he blamed me for the loss of his job and for not being able to drive. He was right; but I couldn't face another disaster.

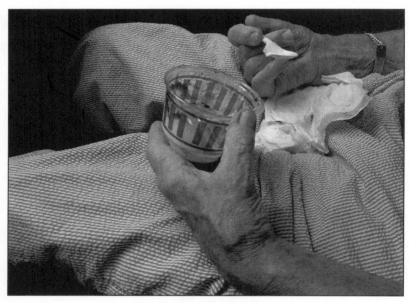

Ken eating ice cream
Philadelphia June, 2010

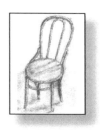

CHAPTER SEVEN

The move to Queens to live in an apartment in our son Ed's house and to be near his family will always be another mystery to me. Our daughter Margie and her husband Edwin drove us there. We arrived at a three story row house with a front porch on a wide street with dark brick houses lined on both sides. Inside, another long set of steps led us up to the second floor apartment. It was pleasant and bright and felt familiar, the high ceilings and large rooms similar to those in my childhood house on Charles Street in Pittsburgh. Three large windows faced a small backyard. When I looked out, I couldn't see much but the backs of other houses until I looked up and saw the sky, bright in the afternoon sun. There were sheets hanging on a line a few row-houses down. I liked looking at all the laundry lines that people had in their backyards, looping from one building to the next, a melody of colors from the clothes hanging on them. Ed told us how badly the apartment had been damaged by the former tenants, and I could see that he had done a lot of work to get it to look as good as it did.

Margie and Edwin again came and helped us. They painted the kitchen, brought us some cooking utensils and generally did everything they could think of to help us manage the new situation. The realization that the family cared about what happened to us helped me to shake myself out of my depression and I began to think, to focus.

I immediately started decorating. Much of the stuff from our life in Edgewood was in boxes on the floor of the dining room. I found one of my favorite objects, a silver metal pitcher, and placed it on the wide windowsill. It was a traditional shape, one bulbous lower part coming to the top with a generous curve and out again to define the top rim, the slender handle reaching from the top down to the middle of the bulb.

I put my painting easel in the window area, even though I knew that in my disheveled state of mind I wouldn't be painting for while. I decided right then and there I would start working on my first memoir about life in Pittsburgh again.

I needed to think seriously about Ken's state of mind, to reassess his mental and physical state, to figure out how to explain his behavior to myself and others, and how to deal with it. I had more or less ignored him during all of the turmoil about selling the house and moving. Ken helped to clean out the Edgewood house, talked to Jim when he was there and gave him a lot of his woodworking tools, but had little to say to me. He watched the workers when the drains had to be replaced, but referred all of their questions to me. He didn't hear when people spoke to him.

He lost track after the first few words, and his attention span was extremely short, another sign of dementia that could also be a result of his depression.

I didn't have the time or the patience to do more than help with his basic needs. I had a hard time figuring out my own actions. As always with me, I tend to be intuitive. Knowledge rattles around in my brain until I need it, and then I have to get to work to put it together sequentially, so that it can be useful.

Dementia is like a virus on the computer. It sneaks in and you don't know about it until it knocks out the other systems. All of these little things that were going on suddenly added up to one big thing: Ken couldn't concentrate, he couldn't do things that require planning, he couldn't focus, because he couldn't remember! Sudden actions, too many demands or directions, caused confusion. Too many alternatives presented, too many questions, or more than one question, did the same. Almost every situation was new to him and he didn't want to be wrong. His reaction was not just confusion, but frustration at questions about what he was doing. He had to work hard to focus on the activity he was involved in and questions or directions were an intrusion. To get him to hear and understand what was being said, I had to ask him to sit down, or put down whatever he had in his hands. Then I had to wait till he was ready, then talk to him about one thing at a time. Normal pace was too fast for him. He was unpredictable; his "operating" system had crashed.

Ken's physical state was in need of attention, too. He needed help to stay healthy. His deteriorating mental state was sometimes predicated on lack of energy, depression, pain from arthritis, infections from neglected tooth decay. I monitored his medications, saw that he got to doctor's appointments, went places with him a few times a week and let him go on his own when it seemed relativity safe.

I needed to understand his reality. I couldn't really know what he was thinking, but I could sense what he understood and what confused him. I forced myself to be patient when he seemed confused or not really aware of what was happening around him. Sometimes I thought of that old cliché, "My heart aches for him.", and wondered if he was he lonely behind that impassive face? Maybe he thought of me as the enforcer rather than the partner? Was he angry and confused about the move to New York? No doubt I was projecting my own feelings. Maybe he just couldn't get over the anger and confusion of all these transitions.

I missed his companionship and the pleasant things he used to say. I missed the closeness of working something out together. "Do you remember the time you built shelves in the kitchen for the new dishes? " I asked. "No," he said, "did I really?" "Yes, in Edgewood. I painted them white and they looked great. When we put the dishes, a whole new set, on the shelves we stood back admiring our work and suddenly all the shelves pulled out from the wall and all of the dishes smashed on the floor! It was so spectacular it was funny and we laughed and laughed!" How hard it was for me to accept that this small piece of our history was lost to him.

It seems that all we did was go to doctors. Beth Israel Medical Center, recommended to us by the cardiologist at University of Pittsburgh, was in Manhattan, which was a long way from Queens. Finding our way in New York City was not easy. There were no buses from our part of Ridgewood, Queens so we had to use the subway. Ken was used to hopping into a car and got very impatient with going up and down stairs constantly, and the long walk to the station from either direction. He refused to believe he'd be cold waiting on subway platforms, and it was impossible to convince him to dress warmly without an argument.

After the initial heart assessment made by Dr. Kalman, the head of the Cardiology at Beth Israel Hospital in New York, Ken was given prescribed Coreg, a medication that would strengthen his heart muscle. A few weeks later he did seem to have more energy and less depression. Daily walks helped and he began to enjoy them instead of just trudging along with me.

Then another challenge presented itself. His poor health had exacerbated the problems he had always had with his teeth, causing one infection after another. Poor teeth and lack of daily oral care cause other infections to flare up and can affect the heart function. What might have been, in a healthier person, a minor ailment became a major emergency. We tried to get help in New York, went to the dental clinic and were told that his condition was too serious and they would not accept him as a client.

As caretaker, it was important for me to understand various ways for Ken to avoid getting more tooth and mouth infections. After weeks of monitoring him, I was able to get him accustomed to using soap when he washed his hands. I refused to go out with him unless he stopped picking pennies up from the sidewalk - " But they're my lucky pennies" he would say. I asked him repeatedly to throw away tissues after he used them. He would remember what I asked him to do for a while and then would go back to the old habits. I realized I was becoming his short-term memory with my constant reminders.

The phone was another problem. He couldn't learn how to use it to make calls; it completely baffled him. I was upset at first, but said little. At least he could answer it, and that saved a lot of anxiety for both of us. I realized I couldn't keep a leash on him. I didn't want him to go out and get lost or get hurt, but I had to be reasonable about it. I further realized that he was going to do whatever he wanted to do and would sneak out if I told him he shouldn't go out for reasons like icy sidewalks or high temperature. I never did quite solve that one.

I tried reason. "If you stay here till I come back we can then go wherever you need to go," I would promise. That tactic worked pretty well.

I began to pay more attention to Ken. We started investigating the shopping area several blocks away, stopping for coffee or lunch. I asked him questions about all of this moving around, what he thought of it. His answer was almost always: "It's OK." I understood how he must have felt. Our life in Pittsburgh had become so stressful, I have to believe that he wanted to get away too, but he couldn't make that choice. I made the choice for both of us. I needed to be patient and listen to him and believe that it was OK. It made me feel sad sometimes, but I was quite sure that I could not have stayed much longer in that situation.

Ken wasn't the only problem occupying me in those days. Terry wrote saying that she was managing. She always seems to be optimistic that the latest place, treatment center or situation, was going to work. I wondered if she was finding it easier to live in such a structured situation, felt safer. I asked Ken to read the letter and tell me what he thought about it. "She always stonewalled," he said. I asked him what that meant to him. "She never slowed down until she got what she wanted."

I couldn't get him to say more about it. I asked him if he would like to read some of my journal notes about what had been happening in our family over the past few years and talk about some of them. He read them very quickly. I think he did not understand them. His only comment was that he liked the quote from the Rabbi Twerski, spiritual leader, author, and former director of a drug clinic in Pittsburgh, about the definition of spirituality: "All the unique features of a human being in their totality is what constitutes the spirit of a person. When an individual exercises these unique features, he or she is being spiritual."

Ken and I talked about spirituality for a while, something that we had seldom done before. I believe in what Rabbi Twerski said and Ken believes in it, too. We demonstrate our spiritually in different ways. Ken believes in prayer, heaven, and the Catholic dogma. I think about today and living in the world. We are loving to each other and our family and try to be kind and considerate to our friends. Ken always gave money generously to our family members when they needed it, and cheerfully donated to many charities throughout his life.

At Ed's house in Queens we soon established a routine. After breakfast I would do needed cleaning in the apartment. Then we did shopping, walked to the library or went into Manhattan for Doctor's appointments. In the afternoon we sometimes got to see our grandchildren, Jack, who was seven, and Sadie, who was four. That was the nicest part of the day.

When Ed asked us to move into the upstairs apartment in his house I knew that he and his wife Merin were unhappy, but I did not realize that the marriage was already on the rocks and that Ed and Merin were in the process of splitting up. Merin and the kids lived in the apartment on the first floor. Ed was living in the basement. Ed seldom came upstairs to visit us; in fact he was seldom around.

Merin did not talk to us much at all. She would usually let the kids come up to visit for a while every day after she picked them up from school. They would talk or watch television, but never stayed for very long. Once a week I made dinner for Merin, Jack, and Sadie.

When it was decent weather, I could hear Jack and Sadie playing in the backyard and that was friendly and comforting. They were very quiet and well behaved, and never talked about Ed with us. I knew that their behavior reflected the conflict going on between their parents and the grief and confusion they felt. My heart broke for them, but I did not know what to do. In many ways, our hands were tied. We were late- comers to the situation, and strangers in New York. It was an unhappy time for all of us.

Ken complained that we never saw Ed. He could sense the atmosphere but made no comment about it until I told him that Ed and Merin were separating and the house was going up for sale. Then he said that he missed seeing Ed and didn't like New York, the first time he made a comment about how he felt about any of our wanderings.

Ed sold the house in Queens in July 2004. The closing was scheduled for September, almost exactly a year from when we had sold our house, and left our familiar world. I could not think about how hard this was for Ed and how anxiety ridden he must have been. He had lost his job, his house, and was now losing his family.

Ken and I had spent two weeks at Margie and Edwin's house in Philadelphia when they went on vacation that summer, and Ken seemed content there. Would this time be the charm? I was hopeful that this might be the last trek.

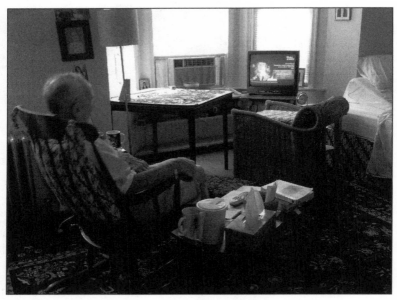

Ken in his room
Philadelphia September, 2012

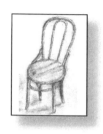

CHAPTER EIGHT

The two weeks in July, 2004 that Ken and I stayed at Margie and Edwin's house in South Philadelphia while they were on vacation in Italy was really the beginning of our move there. We paid the rent for the New York apartment through September, but spent most of the summer in Philadelphia. I felt safe there, but it took a long time to get adjusted.

Unlike Pittsburgh, South Philadelphia is flat land, and much easier to walk than the steep hills we left back home. For the first time since we left Vandergrift 15 years earlier, we again had a walking life. Margie and Edwin's house is nestled in a traditional neighborhood, with easy access to local shops. The grocery store, the library and the church are only a few blocks away. The subway is a block and a half, the buses only a block; the excellent major medical center, Thomas Jefferson University Hospital, is a 10 minute cab ride. In Philadelphia, even without a car, Ken and I became independent again. We went out everyday.

After a few months, I thought it was important to see our extended family and our children Jim and Terry again. Maybe it would encourage familiar memories for Ken to carry with him in our new life. I talked to Ken about possibly visiting his brothers, and he agreed that he wanted to go. He still got confused when presented with alternatives, forgot most things that were said to him, and his judgment was almost nil. I was apprehensive about another move and needed to slow down a bit.

On the way to Pittsburgh I lost Ken in the Philadelphia airport. I asked him to sit down while I waited in the long security line, and when I went back for him he was gone. I panicked, thinking of the thousands of people in the airport, but when I got to a security station, there he was sitting in a chair, patiently attended to by a uniformed security agent. As I was thanking the agent, Ken offered to let a passing girl sit on his lap. It was a shock. In the years I knew Ken, he was always respectful of me around other women. When I tried to explain to him how embarrassing this was to me he didn't answer. I thought: "Do I ever want to travel anywhere with him again?" I doubted it. Ken wasn't embarrassed, even though he would never have done those things before he started on this downward trend. I knew that I would have to find a way to help him slow down and stop inappropriate behavior. If I didn't help him to control these impulses, I couldn't deal with it, and nobody else would tolerate it either.

Our son Jim and daughter-in-law Cindy picked us up at the airport. We stayed in their house perched on a mountaintop outside of Ford City, in the foothills of the Allegheny mountains, about 35 miles from Pittsburgh. Jim and Cindy are easy hosts. They didn't expect much from us, fed us regularly, had lots of books for us to read and understood our habit of sitting around reading and discussing one of Jim's favorite subjects – history. Jim kindly drove us around to see all of the relatives, lengthy trips through western Pennsylvania to see Ken's brother and sister in law, Gene and Thelma, and her family; and to Greenville, where Ken's brother John and Annie lived, and then back to Pittsburgh to visit my sisters Betty and Margie, and of course Terry.

My sister Margie spent a lot of the visit telling me again how much she missed me and the weekly Sunday morning breakfasts. My sister Betty was sick and now living in a nursing home, where she missed my company too. Jim was out of a job and in danger of losing his house. He took us to see Terry at the halfway house where she was now living. Going to see her there was one of the hardest things I ever did. I was numb. Many, many years ago when our son Jim had to go to court I sent Ken. But the time was long past that he would be able to help. When I was a girl, I used to imagine my father in jail for drunkenness, and was upsetting to focus on that memory for even a few seconds. Now, Terry said that she was OK, that she was learning self-discipline and it would last this time. I hoped she was right. She is courageous, but she did look like she had been crying when I came in.

A few days after our arrival at Jim's, Ken missed a step walking into the kitchen. He fell and hit his head against a counter top and was bleeding profusely from a large gash on his skull. Jim and Cindy had gone out for groceries, so in a panic I called an ambulance. I thought about Ken's sister Mary Catherine who had developed dementia after a heart problem, fell when she was at her brother's house, went to the hospital and died there shortly after. Jim and Cindy arrived at the same time as the ambulance, and kept me from a complete melt-down by acting as if it was an every day event. Of course I know that they were not really calm, but their demeanor was very supportive of me and I appreciated it. Ken did not seem to suffer any other bad effects from the fall, and we continued to visit other relatives for a few more days. The incident, how-ever, made me aware that Ken's lack of judgment, a definite symptom of dementia, kept him from relating to the environ-ment and avoiding things that had become unexpected, like steps.

Our visit to Ken's brother Gene and his wife Thelma was especially hard for me. Gene had suffered a massive heart attack several years before when he was still working as a hospital CEO. He worked for a year or two after that, then retired when he began to show signs of dementia. For the five years before his death he became completely dependent on his wife, Thelma; more so than Ken depended on me.

Their six children lived in various parts of the country and were busy with their own lives. So in 2005 Gene and Thelma sold their family house in Washington, Pennsylvania and bought a new, smaller house in a community which offered access to assisted living facilities and nursing home care if needed.

I was upset by Gene and Thelma's decision to buy this house. It felt to me like a withdrawal from the life of the younger world, all old people in neat little homes with all of the conveniences. It felt strangely isolated. It reminded me of movies about the future and robotic living. Maybe it was because we had been somewhat close to making a decision like that ourselves, and I felt like I had just barely escaped it and had dragged Ken with me to safety.

Looking back, I think it is possible that Gene also had Vascular Dementia too. Like Ken, his condition developed a few years after he had a heart attack, but his condition was never diagnosed.

I am still afraid of being lonely. In earlier times people had to live with relatives, they had no place else to go. After the Great Depression, assisted living and nursing homes became a popular alternatives to taking care of elder family members at home. With post World War II new American wealth, the exodus to the suburbs, and the mobility of cars, working class people had become middle class and made choices that were not available to former generations.

My mother's generation knew what it was like living with family but didn't want to burden their children with the idea that they had to be taken care of. I was aware that parent child relationships can become very difficult; expectations from both parties can become burdensome to everyone involved. I believed my children when they offered refuge. But I wanted to live some kind of life of my own.

I had been lonely at Ed's house in Queens. It was only the grandchildren that kept me from that feeling, and the week they were gone on vacation was very lonesome. All of that thinking was leading me toward staying with Margie and Edwin. It sounded like home and family.

When Margie and Edwin returned from their Italian vacation, we sat down to discuss a more permanent arrangement. When I reflect back on it, I think Margie realized long before I did that we would not be able to stay at Ed's. She frequently visited Ed and was more present in Ed's life during the years after we returned from Indonesia than we were. They always had been close, and she saw the trouble brewing on the horizon. Margie and Edwin had bought the house in South Philadelphia with us in mind, and all of this was probably unfolding as she expected, even though it would involve big emotional adjustments for all of us.

Did I want to be cared for? No. I wanted my own house, but I needed help. Ken was complaining about moving around too much. I was glad he was saying it, instead of me wondering how he about it.

We went back to Queens to see what furniture we would like to have in Philly, and this time I was the one who got confused. I left Ken to go to the ladies room at New York Penn Station and when I got back couldn't find him. I suddenly felt like Ken must have been feeling most of the time, disoriented and anxious. I mentally checked off a landmark in the area before I left him, but every part of the station looked the same on the way back. I was near panic when I finally found him sitting right where I had left him. He did better than I did on that one. He just said "Hi, Annie", he didn't even realize that I was gone. If he did, he would have come looking for me for sure.

We did travel back together to New York twice more, once that same November to watch our grandson, Jack, play soccer. He made two goals and Ed said they were the first ones he had made that year. The weather was relatively warm and it felt wonderful. I remember sitting on the grass that felt so soft, like a carpet. There were children running around and playing everywhere. Jack was ecstatic about the goals and Sadie was having fun running around peeking into the big orange plastic cones used to identify the limits of the field. I think this memory helps to mitigate the sadness I felt about leaving my grandchildren, and times we might have spent together.

Again, I don't remember much about the move to Philadelphia from Queens, but this time I had less anxiety. Margie and Edwin were taking care of it and probably had more worries about us than we did about them. The house was being renovated and was still under construction. The first contractor mismanaged the job, including things like pounding nails through plumbing pipes and other horrors. They hired a second contractor who was good, but slow. This time was stressful for Margie, and Edwin was traveling a lot for work and was often gone all week. When I reflect back now, I see that I was once again lost in my own world and didn't pay much attention to what was happening.

Ken and I didn't keep much of our stuff, but the dining room table and the painted wooden hutch Ken had made years ago were too important to leave in Queens. We hung on to some of Ken's woodworking tools, household supplies, a few books and my painting supplies. He was never able again to use the woodworking tools and eventually gave them to Ed and Edwin. I left a lot of things in Queens that I missed for a while, but it was too hard to make decisions about them at the time, and soon it didn't matter.

I felt safe and comfortable at Margie and Edwin's almost immediately, even though the house renovation was far from over. They gave us the second floor, two large bedrooms and a large bathroom. Their bedroom and office were on the third floor, which was originally planned as office space. The three story house, built in the 1880s, was well preserved and cared for, with similar rows on both sides of the wide street. Everything about the street and the houses felt familiar, reminded me of the neighborhood where I grew up on Charles Street in Pittsburgh. On the first night after we returned from that last trip together to New York City I opened the window in Philadelphia and listened to the city sounds: a siren in the distance, a car door slammed shut. I fell asleep feeling like I was in my childhood home on Charles Street.

Even though I felt comfortable and safe, I was not ready to give up my idea of a house of our own. Having a house is essential to living; this is a fundamental belief that has stayed with me throughout my life. Ken and I bought a house when we were first married and it seemed to Ken that owning a house was part of marriage. I remembered one of the comments that he had made many times when we were younger: "The last nail in your house is the first nail in your coffin." Maybe that's why, in what seems now like a confused effort to do something that I felt was important to him, and to me, we went by train to look at houses across the river from Philadelphia in New Jersey. I was appalled by the suburban spread, the highways, the flimsy, cheap houses that were selling for $180,000 - a lot of money at the time and significantly more than our house in Pittsburgh had sold for. The trip eliminated any of my doubts about living with Margie and Edwin.

It hasn't always been easy. Margie and Edwin were stressed and sometimes bickered with each other. One day I told them that I was frightened by their arguing and did not feel comfortable living with them because I was afraid that they would divorce. To their credit, they began to see a counselor the following week. In retrospect, I think that was the beginning of my being able to adjust to this new life with them. My worries about myself and my concerns about being a burden to Margie and Edwin had to take a back seat.

But I felt like a stranger in a strange land, a ship adrift without an anchor. It is hard to let go of old ideas of home. It is even harder to accept that nothing will ever be the same. Ken was not the same person that he had been when he made that comment about the "last nail" years ago at the beginning of our marriage. The man I married will never again be the man I married. I was still in pursuit of something that I thought Ken wanted, when I had no way of knowing his thoughts now. When finally I said to him that I didn't want to leave Philly he surprisingly said, "Neither do I!" I had to face the New Jersey trip for what it was – a whistle in the dark.

I had stopped keeping a journal when we began to leave Edgewood. I didn't want to record what was happening, I just wanted to get through it. My lapse of memory was pretty thorough until a year or so after we arrived in Philadelphia. Margie and I had arguments, most of the time about my lack of communication about how I felt or what I was doing. Sometimes I just wanted to cry, but there was nothing I could do about my thoughts and feelings. I had hoarded them for too long to liberate them, and when I tried I couldn't find the words. I started writing again; the only reliable way for me to explore and share my feelings.

We developed a routine in Philadelphia after a few trials and errors. Within a few months Ken was less anxious and we had begun to get into better habits. His lack of memory made him extremely nervous about daily life, but I think our established routine helped life to be more satisfying for him. Many of the activities, such as keeping track of Ken's medicines and doctor's appointments, were ones that I needed to attend to; but he began developing ones himself that were satisfying. He went to a smoke shop about four blocks away several times a week where he smoked his pipe and got to know and like several men there. He also sat in the backyard and smoked and read at night in the nice weather. Unfortunately, he had some severe pain in his throat after some dental work was done and his cardiologist told him to stop smoking because it was a major risk factor for heart attack and stroke, and just not good for someone who was short of breath anyway. He gave up the smoking immediately, and stopped going to the smoke shop. He said that he didn't talk much to the other men there anyway, which might have been true but I know he missed it.

After a try at Annunciation parish, the closest Catholic church in our South Philly neighborhood, Ken decided for himself that he would like to go to a friendlier one, which was a surprise. As I said before, Ken was always affable, but did not easily engage people. He liked the people he worked with but did not socialize with them otherwise. He never 'hung out' with neighbors, even in Edgewood, which was an intimate community. I know he had friends in college, because I met some of them before we were married, but his brothers were the ones that he talked and laughed and joked with. When we were newly married, I tried to get him to go to neighborhood socials but after one or two of them he refused to go again. During the 1960s and 1970s in Vandergrift, we were outsiders in a small town with an established social pattern, and were not invited. By then, I didn't care. I needed my own friends and found them by working and socializing with my co-workers.

Margie suggested that Ken switch to St. Rita's, a once grand Catholic church not much further than Annunciation, where the priests come out and greets people after the Mass. It feels like a local parish and Ken liked that. He had a sense of community there, and many of the other regular attendees greeted him, too. They asked him how he is doing, and he left with a smile.

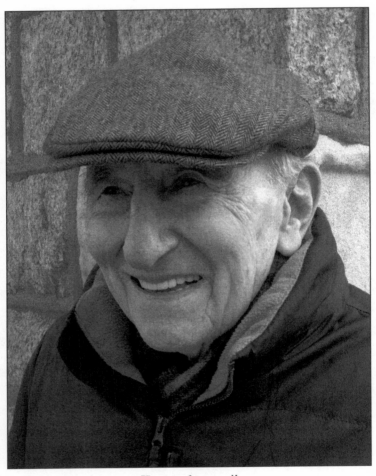

Ken out for a walk
Philadelphia December, 2013

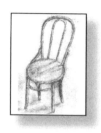

CHAPTER NINE

One day after Sunday mass I asked the pastor at St. Rita's if religious counseling was available, and he recommended Father Mike, a pleasant man with dark hair and beard and warm brown eyes. Father Mike had severe arthritis, which has disabled him since childhood. He seemed to genuinely like Ken, and has been kind to him. Father Mike introduced Ken to St. Therese of Lisieux, who wrote books about living spiritually "in a small way" with day to day prayers. Father Mike seemed to understand Ken's spiritual needs. He listened to him and gave him spiritual books to read. I think these meetings have been some of the most calming and life enhancing experiences that have happened to Ken since we began this journey from our old settled life. Farther Mike extended a genuine welcome to him. Dementia makes people less able to interpret the environment or express their feelings, and talking to Fr. Mike was a large part of Ken's route to finding serenity.

Throughout his life, Ken went to church regularly but did not get involved in either church or school activities. We seldom discussed religion, but he insisted our children go to Catholic School. I was never happy in the Catholic school I had attended, and was not eager to send our children for catholic education. I was surprised Ken was insistent, since he had gone to public school all of his life never attended a catholic school. I had drifted away from the church and its rituals while our children were still young, but I wanted to be tolerant of his beliefs. It was only much later, as the dementia tightened it's hold on his personality, that I began to understand that Ken's spirituality had become a dominant force in his life, and I needed to tend to that aspect of his life as well.

In Philadelphia, Ken would jump up from the dinner table before anyone else finished dinner and shamble directly to his room. Margie suggested that might like to say the blessing before the evening meal. It allowed him to feel more at home in surroundings that were still unfamiliar because of his limited memory, and he was willing to stay a few minutes longer after he had eaten. I found it annoying at first, but I accepted that offering a blessing was an aspect of his religious expression – like saying the rosary every night at 9:30 with the nuns on the Global Catholic Television Network – that filled his daily life with meaning. Saying the rosary became so important to him that he would not watch anything else on TV at that time, even interrupting his favorite ball games to flip the channel to the catholics.

Ken often told us he wanted to "feel useful", and for several of the years that we lived in Philadelphia, he contributed around the house in many ways. One of the first jobs he tackled was the living room fireplace, which Margie had discovered was black slate underneath a hundred years of paint, and wanted to restore it back to the Edwardian original. Ken offered to clean it, a long tedious job. Margie found the right paint remover for the job and Ken spent one or two hours every day for a month or more patiently removing it with a scraper, cleaning the fine points with a tooth brush, and finally polishing it with lemon oil to a beautiful, blue-grey slate finish. He was proud of the gleaming fireplace.

It was really important for Ken – for both of us actually – to feel that we were being useful. Our lives had to a great degree been defined by work. We didn't socialize much except with family, and we didn't drink. Catholic though Ken is, a Protestant work ethic runs deep in him and his farm rooted family. We found meaning in the separate part of our lives in the workplace, and created meaning at home through care of the family and doing projects together. Ken never minded small jobs, and now was happy to take out trash, sweep the backyard. After supper, he began to put the clean dishes away after they were cleaned in the dishwasher.

I assumed Ken was in a routine where he counted his medicines and would tell me if he needed refills. One month he told me that Coreg, his heart medication, was almost gone. My first response was: "Damn! I thought you counted them." I had to correct myself and say: "I'm sorry. I'll help you count them from now on."

He's not to blame. It doesn't work to lay the responsibility on him. He gets upset and feels bad for a while, but doesn't remember why. The emotion lasts but the precipitating memory of the cause is gone. If I left him angry, that's the emotion that would stay with him. I had to understand where he was mentally and remember that he could not accurately interpret verbal or nonverbal cues, another symptom of dementia that can cause anger and anxiety.

Margie, too, thinks about the problems that might arise by all of us living together and I suspect it's her way of accepting what cannot be prevented or changed. She needed to simply accept her Dad and not lead him. You can guide him in certain directions but it has to be related to what is happening in the moment. If the action is upsetting, I try to prevent it in the future by repeatedly going over the event, what made it upsetting, and avoid that the next time. Most things, like Ken's lack of patience at dinnertime when he eats cookies while waiting for the meal, don't matter. What matters are the things that may be dangerous, like a wanting to shovel snow off the sidewalk, where he could easily fall or suffer another heart attack after strenuous activity.

Excellent medical care after the heart attack had improved Ken's physical health, but Ken's mental condition kept deteriorating. His confusion and memory loss were becoming significant, making him even more anxious about daily life.

Now in 2014, Ken's life is further narrowed down to simple rules and activities he is able to recognize and follow. This requires constant monitoring of medications, fluids, and recognition of his needs. Consistently calm responses to his needs help him control the confusion that threatens to overwhelm him. I struggle to understand which part of his mind is working, and which part is muddled. I also struggle to keep my frustration with the situation in check, not always successfully, when his actions and remarks don't make sense to me.

One of the major problems is to help Ken find activities that would give him some feelings of achievement and "feeling useful" without adding to the frustration that occurs when he is faced with ordinary tasks. For instance, shortly after we moved to Philadelphia he spent a great deal of his time writing numbers in long rows on large paper. I tried to figure out what these numbers meant to him without initial success, but he was finally was able to tell me he was keeping track of the lottery numbers. As I write this, I realize that he was looking for a pattern of numbers that would most likely be a winning combination. Ken was always a 'numbers guy'. He spent much of his engineering career writing test lab reports and making number comparisons. Numbers held a certain kind of magic for him. Perhaps he imagined he was solving a problem that had been part of his job so many years ago. Providing him with the materials to experiment with numbers and patterns maybe helped him to keep his mind alive by activating past memories that were less confusing. Even now, he remembers the day's date and the temperature when he remembers almost nothing else. Back then, I attempted to solve the problem by getting him a lottery ticket every week.

He still kept track of those numbers on that huge piece of paper, then gradually forgot about them when I told him he could watch one number on television every evening. After about a year with no win, he gradually gave up the whole project.

After Ken got tired of playing the lottery, jigsaw puzzles became his primary occupation, and still are. One of his brothers told me how much they all liked jigsaw puzzles when they were younger and gave us some that his brother John had used. They were old and the pieces too soft to hold together, but Ken did show interest, so I bought some new ones at Walmart. That was six or seven years ago, and he is still doing puzzles at the rate of about one a week. When I asked him why he likes them so much, he said that it gives him something to resolve. I was surprised at that insight. It's so easy to take for granted that he lives without being able to solve much. I have found little research on insight in people with dementia, but he was an engineer after all, so perhaps problem solving will probably be the last skill to go.

It took some doing to find the right puzzles. Thousand-piece puzzles confused him rather than calmed him, 300 pieces were too easy. He finally settled on 500 pieces, and I buy them on line, a month's supply at a time. He cannot redo them because the pieces do not fit well, so after one session we give them to a local thrift store. Now I simplify the shopping by buying three or four at a time, once a month online.

One day recently he asked me to help him with one he was having trouble with. I looked at it and realized that the pieces were too small and the colors too similar for him to differentiate between them. Ken had sorted them into piles of about five pieces each, trying to coordinate the colors. I suggested that he throw it away and just start on one of the other new ones he had. "I can't throw it away," he said. "Can't we send it back?" I explained why we could not send something back that was open and used. "Well", he said, "I made 75 piles of pieces and I can figure out how to do it if you help me." "You're good at working them," I said, "but I'm not."

After a little more frowning and insistence that we could send it back, he asked me if we could buy something to place on top of it. I found a large piece of cardboard which covered up the previous one. We opened one of the new puzzles, which had more separate colors. He was satisfied with that. This has continued as a process of Ken being able to work two puzzles at once on his bedroom table. If he gets frustrated with one, he can move the unfinished one to the side (still keeping it in view), and start another one. Sometimes he is able to go back and finish the first one; sometimes he pulls it apart and puts it back in the box for a later try. I am continually amazed, and grateful, that this small amount of control over his 'work' has enabled him to be busy and content for years.

In early 2011, Ken started to leave his pajamas on until dinnertime. Margie had bought him a pair of very soft, warm ones for Christmas and maybe he just hated to take them off. I tried teasing him about it at first. When there was no response to that, I suggested it made others uncomfortable to see him in his pajamas all day. When that didn't work, I tried trickery. I asked him to walk to the corner store a few times each week for something we needed before lunch. I also reminded him that the doctor had told him to walk about 15 minutes three or four times a week, which is about how long it takes to go to the store and back.

We live close to public transportation, and far enough from a major highway that you can walk for blocks without crossing a busy street. I walked with him a few times until he got over any confusion about the route. This was one of those decisions I worried about. There is always a risk, but he wanted to do it and I think that once the habit was established, it gave him confidence and a feeling of independence. (He also wears an ID bracelet that has his name, address and my phone number on it, and carries a Jitterbug easy- call phone with him in his pocket. I try not to think about what might happen, but still…). His walks reminded him to get dressed appropriately. I've learned that the major strategy for coping is to keep the goal in mind. All too often, caregivers try to fix everything and end up exhausted and frustrated. It's hard to accept you can't fix this, but that is the truth. You cannot can't make everything all right, and adjustment of goals to be realistic and attainable is not only helpful, it is survival.

Ken's pride in his appearance helps him in other ways. He was a college soccer and tennis player, well centered in his physical and athletic abilities and connected to his physical awareness. As I said before, he always dressed well and took good care of his clothes. He never wanted me to buy clothes for him, even socks. He didn't buy clothes often but the ones he did buy were good ones. He played tennis regularly and kept in shape. Even now, he will watch his consumption of desserts if he thinks he has gained weight, and wears a frayed old belt so he can 'measure' his weight by the belt hole. We can always appeal to that pride if he forgets to take showers, thinks it's OK to wear underwear for three days in a row, forgets to change pajamas, doesn't want to change a favorite shirt, or doesn't realize that his pants have food stains on them. Also, he now reminds me when he needs a haircut, although unfortunately his hair grows shabby long before he recognizes the need for one.

Ken's room has a large bay window, which provides lots of light and a view of the front street, which he ignores. His attention is focused entirely on what is happening with him at the moment. He has a large table in front of the window for his current jigsaw puzzle, a chair covered with cushions to ease the hours he spends there, his back turned away from the rest of the world in the house. Before he sits down, he turns on "Easy Listening" music channel on television, usually a constant stream of the music and songs of the 1940s and 1950s. He never misses a Lawrence Welk show, and listens to the same kind of music on a cassette recorder to help him sleep at night. It's unusual to walk into his room and not hear it playing, softly at night and louder during the day. There has been research done on the effects of music and its effect on the brain but there seems to be little I have found on how it affects dementia. I think music serves as a powerful recollection of those days when Ken was a teenager, the radio was played constantly, the Hit Parade offered a steady diet of the popular swing music and the big bands that played it.

Television confuses him. He usually cannot follow the story line of any program, so watches few movies and no series, which would require remembering prior episodes. The Catholic rosary on TV every night satisfies his spiritual needs and establishes a predictable routine. He also likes to watch baseball all summer, but only if the Phillies are playing. Luckily they play often during the season and he can talk about the game with Edwin, our son-in-law, who makes a real effort to watch TV with him and talk stats.

Phillies baseball is the only sport that Ken watches about which he seldom says: "This is a repeat." It's a remark that he makes about almost anything that he sees, from television sports games to a passerby on the street. It may simply be déjà vu, an experience of having seen or experience something before. I wonder at times if it is because he pulls up something similar from his memory. Or, perhaps it's a phrase he uses because he doesn't recognize the experience and is a cover up for his lack of understanding. So far, I have not found anything in my research about that particular phenomenon.

I go with him to church, to the doctor, and to other places, such as the library, where he has to cross a busy street. He walks very slowly because he gets short of breath and the 15 seconds allowed by the stoplight to cross the four lanes of Broad Street leaves him stranded in the middle. The doctor's office is in Center City. It used to require a bus ride, a walk of three blocks and then two more blocks to the office when we got off the bus. But now in 2014, the shortness of breath is very debilitating and we have to take a cab or be driven wherever Ken goes. A wheel chair seems to be out of the question. Ken refuses to use one, and never complains about how long it takes, or how painful it is, to walk. He understands that as long as he can move, he can be relatively independent. Ken restricts his walk up the flight of stairs to our suite on the second floor to only a few times of day. I have gradually created a "kitchenette" in the small connecting room between our bedrooms and the bathroom with a microwave, an electric teapot and a small fridge. Ken eats his breakfast there, and often makes coffee throughout the day. It has worked pretty well, and has definitely extended his energy and ability to stay in the house.

The subway was our first travel alternative when we moved here because it's only two blocks away. Even though there are steps, there is a place to sit down out of the weather and we are closer to the doctors' offices when we get off. The other advantage of the subway was that we get off in the underground mall and stop for lunch or coffee going or coming. He liked that. It was always part of the routine when we took trips. No matter how far away, his first thought was where we would stop for coffee, or a treat. It's sad to me that we take so many fewer trips together. Now, we seem to fatigue quickly and can't wait to get back home.

Ken has a cell phone for emergencies but has been unable to master making calls. We got him the Jitterbug, a much simpler phone, but he couldn't adjust to the simplicity. It took several weeks for him to realize that he only had to open it to answer. I remind him that you don't have to punch any numbers, just open it up. My name is the first one that comes up when he opens it and he can call me. Even that skill has to be reinforced at least every two weeks or so.

About two years ago, Ken went back to smoking his pipe. One day we asked him what was his favorite thing to do and he said "having a smoke." Margie rummaged around in the cellar and found the box of his pipes that thank goodness we had not thrown away. He was delighted with the recovery of his pipes and immediately went out to the backyard to fire one up. During that summer he smoked outside almost every night, in the sturdy chaise lounge that Edwin bought for him to relax in. Edwin is a dedicated gardener, and the back yard walled garden is a lovely peaceful spot. The times in the garden seem full of contentment for Ken. I sometimes watch him from the kitchen window, watching the birds perch in the ginko tree, studying shifting could patterns as the pipe smoke curls around his face. Even our cardiologist agreed that at the age of 91, quality of life trumps concerns about smoking damaging his health.

Smoking in the winter, when it is too cold to sit outside became the problem. When we first moved to Philly, Ken was able to walk to the near by smoke shop. Years later, he can't walk there and they are not as hospitable to an elderly man who has struggles to breathe, leans on a cane to walk and is a fall risk. When Ken began to smoke again two years ago, we utilized our Long Term Care health policy to hire a companion caregiver to drive him to a smoke shop two days a week. Now we have a new caregiver, and she drives him to the local senior center where he can smoke outside, socialize a bit, and also have lunch. But as I write this, winter is approaching and again we are searching for an indoor safe harbor for Ken the pipe smoker. He asks us about it every day; finding a good place to smoke is one of his final concerns in life. He has little olfactory stimulation in terms of taste and smell from years of sinus infections, so smoking is one of the most pleasurable aspects of his life – along with the nightly bowl of ice cream.

I have long since taken over control of the money. This transfer of power was difficult in some ways for me. I had always had a certain amount of control over decisions about the children, but not dealing with money. He insisted on paying all of the bills each month, even if it meant we had less than I felt we needed for food and I felt that some bills could be partially paid or left for another month. He spent hours every month balancing the checkbook. The only way to relieve him from worrying about the money was to earn some myself. My solution then was to work part time. Now, my solution is to dole out dollars for certain things.

We still stop for coffee after doctor's visits, go out for lunch once a week or so. I now fill his church envelopes and leave dollar bills in a box where he can get them. He gives it all away, to church, to any charity that asks for it, to people on the street that beg for it. He will not keep any for himself, except to get his haircut. He complains about the price of that, and we have to remind him that it is not 1950 anymore. I'm not sure he believes us. To him maybe it is.

He asks for books, starts reading and in a few hours announces that he has finished it. He reads the words but, if we ask him, does not know what he read or he says that he had read it before. He is aware that something is wrong, but I think he makes it all right in his mind by covering up his lack of memory.

He wears a mask of sorts. One of the first things he does in the morning is read the bible. Many of the other books he reads are on religious subjects and these he reads over and over, sometimes making the comment that he doesn't understand them, sometimes picking out a particular passage to read out loud.

Now, in 2014, Ken is seemingly no longer aware of what he used to be. Is this a blessing or a curse? I still wonder.

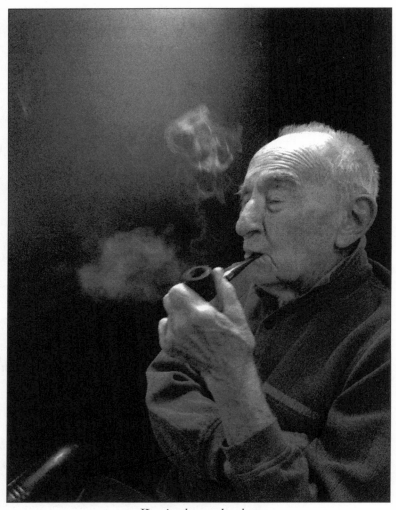

Ken in the smoke shop
Philadelphia February, 2014

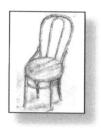

CHAPTER TEN

My life has always been shaped by the necessity of care giving. When my mother worked the night shift scrubbing floors at a local hospital in Pittsburgh, my sister and I had to take care of our younger brother and sisters.

I have a lasting memory of my father sitting in our living room on Charles Street, one dark trousered knee crossed over the other, eyebrows like bristly wings protecting his dark brown eyes, reading the encyclopedia or the newspaper, stopping in the middle of a murmured Irish tune to greet me with a soft grunt. When I was twelve, I knew that I loved him. But by the time I was sixteen I was ashamed of him, and no longer knew whether I loved him or not. Why did he drink so much that he turned into a different person; one who raged instead of singing, one who stormed about the house instead of reading? It puzzled me, and made me sometimes fear him. Now, at age eighty eight, I wonder if my mixed emotions about his moods and his inability to function when he was drinking led me to a fascination with psychiatry, to eventually practice psychiatric nursing, and sustained my interest in Ken's dementia.

In 1945, when I was eighteen and began training at St. Joseph's School of Nursing on the South Side of Pittsburgh, I knew nothing yet about psychiatry, but I quickly learned about confused minds and how to alleviate resulting agitation. The Second World War was nearing its end. The Jones and Laughton steel mill in Pittsburgh was still operating at full capacity making basic steel. The men worked hard in a hot, noisy atmosphere and it was customary for them to stop on the way home at one of the numerous saloons on the main street. They and their wives were usually first generation Americans whose parents were immigrants from Eastern Europe. The wives worked hard too, cleaning constantly to keep their small row houses spotless, in spite of the smoke and dirt from the mills throughout the Pittsburgh area.

Most of the men were admitted to the hospital with heart attacks or broken bones or burns from their close proximity to the furnaces. They demanded - and needed - their liquor, becoming angry and combative if they didn't get it. Relatives brought in whiskey which was kept in a locked "whiskey cupboard" on the men's floor of the hospital. The drink was needed to alleviate symptoms of delirium tremens which, I realized many years later, can be similar to dementia symptoms such as confusion, anger, agitation and disorientation.

At nursing school I learned a lot about dealing with difficult patients, education that was useful later when I served on the psychiatric unit at St. Francis Hospital in Pittsburgh. As student nurses there we were required to read the case studies of our psychiatric patients and were expected to apply our knowledge to find a way to communicate with them - to be patient, to listen to them, to understand their body language. This was before the advent of psychiatric medicines, and calmness and a caring attitude were essential. That was not hard for me, as I had been studying body language and the meaning of harsh words and anger for most of my life at home. And I had learned some safe responses when I couldn't hide to avoid the chaos.

When Ken began to be affected by the symptoms of dementia, I found myself becoming a caregiver again. I started out with confidence, thinking that I knew about caring for somebody with difficult mental and emotional problems. I soon found out that I knew less than I thought I did. No matter how much you love someone, being with a person who is slowly becoming unable to function appropriately is stressful and inhibits the caregiver's understanding. If it was hard for me, a nurse who has had experience with those who were mentally and emotionally vulnerable, how must it be for a caregiver who has not had those experiences?

Through all of our married life I had often asked Ken questions about his feelings, and he would refuse to answer. Over the years I had to learn to accept Ken's emotional remoteness. When I talked to him recently about his young life, he said that he did what he was supposed to do, what everybody else was doing. He did what was expected. He said he was unobtrusive, didn't try to get attention, avoided trouble, tried to please people and tried to be a good person. His former view of life is a good indicator of how I understand his current behavior: He waits to be told what to do in many situations, he tries to please at all times, he makes no demands, he believes that he will go to heaven if he is good, helps others and goes to Catholic mass and receives Holy Communion regularly. He believes in the here-after. His prayers fill our house; his spiritual life sustains him.

I grieve for Ken, but I am pursuing my own goals. Always in the back of my mind are worries about my own future.

I need color and beauty. I think I would die from lack of it. Bold, bright colors keep the grey away. I remember a piece of batik I had seen in a store in Indonesia. It enchanted me, and still gives me a pleasurable memory of green and blue, deep blue and light green when I recall it. It was enormously expensive but what a pleasure it would have been to own! I realize now, looking back, that I was looking at a work of art, one as powerful as any painting in a museum that I have ever seen.

When we first moved to Philadelphia, I sewed — a sofa cover, cushions, travel bags for Margie and her friend, Cate, and Cate's daughter, Claire. I made doll clothes for our granddaughter Sadie and for our niece's daughter. The sewing reminded me of the many things I have put together from whatever was available. Getting through. Doing what has to be done. Trying to make beauty.

Sewing prefigured my return to painting, which more challenging work. I decided to sign up for painting classes, realizing happily that I was back on the path to my real goals, painting and writing. Throughout these years, I have continued to paint, and the walls of our house are full of my work. Now I have a new thrill - painting flowers on greeting card stock, which I send to my family and friends. They seem delighted with this gift, and I find endless pleasure in being able to create them.

Years go, when we first moved here to Philadelphia, Margie and Ken and I went out one day to get a cup of coffee and we ended up having an argument about something related to Ken being cold. He refused to wear a sweater, he insisted on getting coffee, then said he didn't want any. I snapped at Margie as well as Ken. Ken's silent, uncomfortable sulking continued in the car on the way home and lingered for days after. For Ken, the unfortunate consequence of anger is that he retains an impression of the emotion and it lasts long after the event. I know that this is a symptom of dementia, and yet I was not able to control my anger at the time. At that moment, I felt like my whole life was a failure. I felt guilty of all kinds of past offenses. I felt stupid that I didn't know these things. I cried and cried that evening and had a hard time stopping. Unfortunately, this is a pattern I continue to struggle with.

No doubt this is another reason that parents have a hard time living with their children. The past rises up to haunt everyone involved. In this instance, when I was able to be rational again, I recognized that I had always trusted Margie and had learned through all of the turmoil to trust Edwin as well. I apologized.

One night in 2008 I woke up after something inside my chest gave a thump. Not a mild one like you might expect from indigestion, but a very strong, determined THUMP, as if someone hit me in the chest. Only vaguely worried at first, I called the cardiologist about it the next day, expecting him to tell me that I was all right, and not to worry. Instead he told me to come in to see him immediately and ordered an electrocardiogram, which indicated that I had suffered a ventricular tachycardia, which is a rapid heart beat that arises from improper electrical activity of the heart. A day later I had a defibrillator implanted in my chest and spent the following three days in the hospital. I had three electrocardiograms each day to make sure I could tolerate the recommended medication, Tikosyn, which the doctor advised could have some worrisome side effects. I wandered around the hospital cardiology department, talked to nurses, read. It was a vacation from my worries and problems. Ken was in good hands with Margie and Edwin. I felt free for a few days, secure in the knowledge that the defibrillator would keep me from dying if my heart stopped again.

Those three days of freedom led me to dreaming of a house of my own again. A place where we, including Margie and Edwin, could go for the summers away from humid Philadelphia, and close enough to Ed that he could take care of it. It would belong to all of us. It seemed so simple at the time.

This led me too the unfortunate decision to use our money from the Edgewood house to make a down payment on a house in the Pocono Mountains, near Ed. Ed had written and published a book of humorous essays called STUPID WARS, and his house repair business was doing well, so he felt confident about taking responsibility for a house, and agreed to make the monthly mortgage payments. Against the advice of Margie and Edwin, I bought the house. Almost immediately after the first few payments the Great Recession of 2008 started and his ability to make the monthly payments plummeted. I had been stalled in that stage of vulnerability that happens after so much emotional turmoil, a terrible time to make more decisions. I was becoming obsessive. I thought I needed a house and nothing would stop me. Even Ken, who I thought was the obsessive one, was more practical and agreed with Margie and Edwin.

I borrowed money to make the payments until the house was sold, which took almost a year. We sold it at a loss, and lost all of the money we had invested, plus that which I had borrowed from our insurance.

Gone was all of my calmness about doing the right thing in leaving our home in Edgewood. Gone was my ability to pay much attention to Ken. Gone was any good humor that I was clinging to. I couldn't think of anything except that this was the worst mistake I had ever made. After we sold the house it took a long time for me to forgive myself. I blamed it on fear of dying, and leaving nothing, and that may well have been true.

Luckily for Ken and me, Margie and Edwin never made an issue of it and did not refer to it or to money at all, the best thing they could have done for me. The only problem was that I cried a lot, again, and Margie was upset that I couldn't explain why. She encouraged me to write my first book, "My Charles Street", a memoir I'd started in Pittsburgh four years before. She edited the book and published it. She continued to encourage my painting, and I gained enough confidence to do more modern painting and eventually sell some of my work.

Ken had moved to a relatively calm state, needing only help with medications, transportation or help getting to church or doctor's visits, coffee or lunch out from the house two or three times a week. Easy, calming things. Terry was calmer, too. She attended Mercy Behavioral Health program in Pittsburgh and we talked by phone several times a week.

After the Pocono Mountain house was finally sold and the only panic left was to pay leftover bills, I found that my perspective on life had undergone another change. I understood I could not control everything in life; in fact very little.

I realized that I was grieving not only for Ken, but for loss of my own home, of having no place to call my own.

Only recently have I begun to understand the reasons why I could not abandon Terry when her drug addiction resulted in her inability to function; that I needed to stay with Ken when his dementia caused a similar disability. I learned this response from my family. My mother did not abandon my father in spite of his alcoholism and disregard for his family's needs. To thrive, people need a home, a place to be completely accepted and comfortable. In our society, those without that security often feel home-less, as if they are not important enough to belong to, or have, a family; that they are being thrown away like an old dishrag.

Losing the Pocono house was a step toward understanding that where I am is my own place, as much as any place else would be. I felt like a coward when we left our Edgewood house in Pittsburgh. But I think now that I was not always running away from a problem, I was running to shelter. Maybe I was always running to safety, like running and hiding in the third floor closet when my mother and father were fighting. I couldn't run away from Ken or Terry, but ran toward help from those who offered it.

Maybe the Pocono house was my last fling at being decisive, but the whole experience gave me a huge scare about being, or trying to be, involved in a new world that was unfamiliar to me. I know something now I didn't know before. I have a harder time understanding so many parts of my world that had always seemed natural before, including one that assured me that I could do whatever I wanted to, if I only try. I simply do not have the abilities to do what was once simple for me. I learned age really does matter.

Now, my optimistic view of that world may be in imminent danger. I have an accumulation of guilt I can't seem to shed and become overwhelmed when I try to talk about it.

And yet, I feel happier than I have ever been. Sometimes the past is the present. As Toni Morrison said: "To be truly at home in the present, we must confront the past." I try to wake myself up to the life around me, to the status of my own emotions, to participation in the lives of others. I think about the source of my creativity and the spirituality I have long denied. I found out that spirituality and faith are is not a set of rituals, but deeply meaningful characteristics of being human and caring for those we love.

Ken is living a life that is satisfying to him. I'm not sure that he understands what he believes, but he has strong spiritual feelings. He does not have much pain and he doesn't remember enough to have much fear. He lives in the moment.

I have no patience with the rituals of religion, but I have my own path. I believe that each human being has a unique essence and that nurturing it, despite our difficulties, is what makes us human.

I do not feel we are a burden to our children. They are ours and we are theirs. When we needed help they responded, as we tried to do for them as they needed and asked for it. In the final assessment, I think we chose well, and chose the happier alternative.

I wrote this book to look back on my life with Ken, to remember and think about what he did and didn't do, what he might have felt and didn't feel. When I think about the motives behind his former behaviors I can see how his actions now are related to those feelings and behaviors from his past. To me, it seemed that his memory loss and confusion mask his identity. Now, at this point in my life, I am left to imagine how he feels and wonder if I ever really knew his real identity.

When Ken developed dementia, I determined that I would do whatever I could to keep that loneliness that had haunted us both from happening to him again.

"Where are my people?" a friend's mother repeatedly asked when she was put into a nursing home. I wasn't sure what I was doing when I became Ken's caregiver, but instinctively I knew I would try to keep his family with him.

KEN'S LETTER

In June of this past summer I had a mild stroke and was in the hospital for a day. This is a letter found on a forgotten page in a notebook on Ken's table many weeks later. I share it with you in the hope that hearing some of his own words you can imagine him more fully.

June 27, 2014

> *Today is the day I would like to start writing.*
>
> *I would like to think of God and Jesus and their help in everyday life. All of the things that are given to us should make us thankful and cooperative in helping others less fortunate than us.*
>
> *Annie came home from the hospital yesterday. She had a "small stroke" in her right eye. She said it was not serious and hopefully no follow-up. The hospital seems thorough and tries to prevent any repercussions.*
>
> *Thanks for the TV, music, pretty girls and sports. What every happened to the baseball season — I'll never know. They show the same games over and over.*
>
> *The jigsaw puzzles help but pieces seem to disappear and I can't find them.*

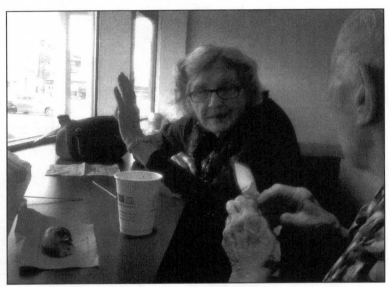

Anna and Ken at the donut shop
Philadelphia April, 2013

COPING: A QUICK LIST

There is no cure for dementia and much of the care for the patient is taken by family members or professional caregivers. Through the years of care giving, I learned how to help Ken use his own body and mind to live with the dementia, and how I could encourage his independence and thus make his own life less stressful. My advice is to get help in any way you can. Demand information from your doctor or therapist, ask about agencies that can help. The Alzheimers Association (www.alz.org, 24/7 Helpline 800.272.3900) has the best information that I found about all stages of dementia, but obviously there are many other resources.

Here are some strategies for coping that helped me as caregiver:

1. Keep the Goal in Mind

Often, caregivers trying to make everything all right will end up exhausted and frustrated. Decide what is realistic and attainable. Controlling risk factors can slow the progress of vascular dementia. Risk factors include high blood pressure, cholesterol, lack of exercise and smoking.

2. Anticipate Misinterpretation

The individual with dementia is not able to accurately interpret verbal or non-verbal cues which can result in anxiety and frustration in both the individual and the caregiver. Try to be clear and concise in your communications, repeating things as needed by using the same words or message. Try to imagine what someone might think or say if they were able to think clearly, and try to respond to what makes common sense. Emotions are often volatile. Anger erupts because he/she may think something opposite to whatever it is that you are trying to explain.

3. Remember Behavior has a Purpose

Many experts believe that some of the behavioral symptoms that people with dementia exhibit, such as shouting out or striking out, are meaningful. Although the person does not generally intend to disrupt things or to hurt someone, they do intend to be noticed and perhaps communicate a need that is not being met. In addition, it is important to remember that while these behaviors are meaningful, they are not intentional. The individual is not doing this "on purpose," but more likely in an attempt to give a message they can no longer explain in words. Slowing down, trying to see the world through their eyes and trying to respond to the 'feeling" behind the behavior rather than the behavior itself, may allow you to prevent an emotional crises and keep life running more smoothly.

4. Reminisce About the Past

Since memories from the distant past are not usually affected, encourage discussions about people and places that are familiar and evoke pleasant feelings for both of you. It can help the person with dementia, and you the caregiver, to continue to feel connected and to contribute.

5. Be Flexible

The disease is progressive. Symptoms and needs will change over time. If strategies are no longer working, don't use them. Seek help, ask for advice; learn from others who have had similar experiences. More challenging behavioral symptoms such as resisting care or depression can be particularly difficult and often require a very individualized approach. Talk to your doctor about approaches, both pharmacological and non-pharmacological.

6. Safety

Providing increasing supervision is a difficult and time-consuming task for many caregivers. In the early stages, reminders and cues in the environment may be enough to keep the person safe. When more supervision is needed it is best to assess each situation individually and gradually increase the amount of supervision needed to maintain as much independence and autonomy as possible in as safe a setting as can be provided. When the person can no longer be cared for at home, a local government agency that supports elder care can be very helpful in guiding you to resources, and the services of a geriatric care manager if appropriate.

7. Establish a Routine

Focus on simplification. Make a list of realistic expectations for the patient:

> a. The amount of exercise he/she can tolerate. This can be determined by the combined efforts of the doctor and the cardiac rehab and/or the rehabilitation therapist.
>
> b. What kind of food he/she needs, how much liquid they should have
>
> c. Serve meals at approximately the same time each day.
>
> d. Do not pamper the person, too much help encourages dependence, he/she becomes dependent because the world has become confusing.
>
> e. Establish a good routine by simplifying his/her life

f. When you ask him/her to help, make the request as simple as possible

8. Offer Simple Choices

Reintroduce activities the person once enjoyed: reading, puzzles, painting, or introduce new ones to have him/her try. The person with dementia often develops habits which may be annoying and seem obsessive compulsive, but actually he/she is trying to order his confusing life.

A FINAL NOTE

There is some recent research evidence that hospitalization can increase the chances of Alzheimer's and Dementia patients moving into a nursing home, or dying, within the year following the hospitalization. The risk is even higher if those patients experience delirium, a state of extra confusion and agitation, during their hospital stay. This is a concept that I intuitively adopted and agree with. I believe that caregivers need to know this risk so they can help a loved one with dementia avoid the hospital if possible.